D1738754

New Approaches in Child Guidance

edited by

Herbert S. Strean

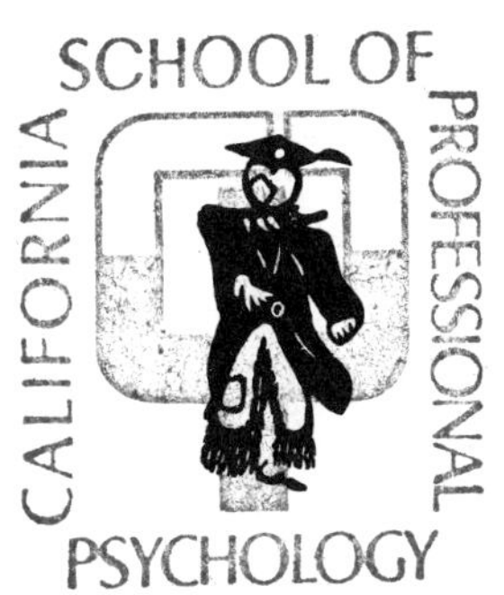

The Scarecrow Press, Inc.
Metuchen, N.J. 1970

ISBN 0-8108-0330-5

Contents

1. Introduction: Rationale and Organization of the Text

by Herbert S. Strean

During the past decade the child guidance movement has witnessed dramatic modifications in its therapeutic modalities and the theoretical perspectives which guide its practice. Originally, the movement was conceptualized as one in which the child was the complete focus of diagnostic and treatment attention; the social worker or child therapist devoted virtually all of his efforts to the understanding and alleviation of the child's intrapsychic conflicts. By the 1940's workers began to recognize that as the youngster made progress in his treatment and functioned with more freedom, this frequently activated anxiety in his mother. Professionals soon realized that a childhood behavior disorder or a childhood neurosis was often, if not always, unconsciously induced and sustained by the mother and modifications in the child's behavior, no matter how positive, adversely affected his mother's equilibrium. Consequently, instead of just presenting their children's social histories and then sitting in the waiting room while their youngsters were being treated, mothers became clients, too. This development appreciably helped the youngster inasmuch as the mother did not have to defeat the child's therapy or the results of it if her own psychosocial needs were being attended to by her own therapist. However, as mother and child improved in their internal functioning and modified their transactions with each other, father often felt excluded by them and became threatened by their changes. Efforts in the 1950's, therefore, tended to include him in the diagnostic and treatment plan.

A natural step in the evolution of the child guidance movement was the realization that the family could be viewed as a social system with interdependent parts; therefore, a change in one part of the system could alter the entire system. Hence, family therapy came into vogue and the child began to be considered more as a symptom or dysfunction of the family system; thus, the entire system needed treatment. The child, although presented as "the problem," was the family's displayed expression of family conflict.

Lately, the child guidance movement has moved into larger orbits--the extended family, the neighborhood, and community. Community mental health units are frequently manned by child guidance workers and the problems that they confront are diagnosed within the framework of a community perspective. A child's school phobia, for example, is now considered more than a problem of "separation anxiety." The professional of today would not discount the child's feeling of anxiety as he separates from his mother, but, in addition, he would also be interested in how the parent-child, parent-parent, husband-wife, family, school, and neighborhood subsystems contribute toward aiding and abetting this problem. Therefore, a youngster with a school phobia in Harlem might call forth differential treatment efforts from one living in Scarsdale. Psychological, social, economic, organizational factors would all be of enormous importance as the child and his situation were diagnosed and treated.

The organization of this book is designed to parallel the evolution of the child guidance movement. The early chapters deal with diagnostic and therapeutic efforts in work with the individual child exclusively. It is followed by chapters on group therapy with children and individual and group therapy with parents. We then move on to a consideration of family diagnosis and family therapy and then turn to the diagnosis of larger social units--institutions and subcultures.

As the practice focus of child specialists has been modified, so have the uses of theoretical perspectives. In the 1940's, child guidance was essentially dominated by Freudian psychoanalysis, a theory which concentrates almost exclusively on the child's internal life and his psychopathology. However, as the youngster's progress in and out of the treatment situation began to be viewed as dependent on his transactions with many significant others, and as child development was gradually conceived as much more than the unfolding of instincts, ego psychology, learning theory, communication, role, systems, organizational theories became relevant in the conceptualizations of childhood problems and their treatment. For example, when the worker concentrated on the family as a unit, the complementarity of family members' roles and their role expectations of each other became salient issues in diagnosing and treating dysfunctional elements in the family system. Now that a "good" family system is seen not so much as consisting of neurotic-free individuals but more as units that do or do not accommodate each other, notions from organizational theory and systems theory have become pertinent.

Although the child guidance specialist now has a flock of theoretical perspectives from which to choose, and despite the fact that he has not sufficiently developed criteria whereby he may extract appropriate concepts and constructs from the various theories, his openness to various perspectives has been an enriching phenomenon in work with children and their parents. One advantage of being able to choose from alternative theoretical perspectives has made the child guidance worker more responsive to the psychosocial needs of the individual client. He can now relate various approaches to the client and his situation rather than fitting the client into one precious theoretical model that must be preserved. This book attempts to demonstrate this receptivity of the child guidance person to new theoretical perspectives. For example, "The Use of the Patient as Consultant" and the chapters on adolescents demonstrate the applicability of role theory and ego psychology to the treatment of childhood disorders. The work of Professor Leonard Brown on the mentally retarded borrows heavily from social systems and role theories and the several chapters on group psychotherapy show the alliance between the child guidance worker and the small groups theorist. Professor Neal Brown's paper demonstrates how several theoretical orientations can be weaved together in the assessment of certain psychosocial problems.

As child guidance personnel have become less wedded to Freudian psychoanalysis as a theory of treatment, the role of the therapist has been considerably modified. The child guidance worker now views himself not solely as a conveyor of interpretations and clarifications but more as a human participant in a transactional process. This transactional process is designed to provide corrective emotional experiences to the client rather than just intellectual insight. The worker now attempts to understand how the client has been deprived of significant human experiences and then offers these experiences in the therapy. The client who has been deprived of limits and structure will be offered limits and structure by the therapist; those who have been deprived of warmth and understanding will be given these ingredients by the therapist; and those who have not had the opportunity of discharging angry impulses will be permitted to do this. This notion of supplying the necessary attitudes and services that have been missing in the client's life is particularly true in social casework where food is provided to the hungry, clothing to the cold and housing to the ill sheltered.

It may be said that virtually every paper in this volume underscores the notion of the corrective emotional experience. Kesten's "Learning Through Spite" demonstrates how a youngster who has been prodded to achieve is given a therapeutic experience where virtually nothing is expected of him; Dr. Colm's paper on phobic children underscores the importance of the therapist's making restitution to children who have been deprived of essential human experiences during the early parts of their lives; and the paper by Rosenthal and Black again reveals this same theme.

As the therapist tunes in to the child and/or parent's emotional life whether it be in individual, group, family or institutional treatment, he is always enacting a role--a role designed to enhance his client's psychosocial functioning. Although a conveyor of interpretations is also a therapeutic role, the contemporary therapist enacts many roles which mirror the whole range of human experience. He offers warmth and coolness, insight and indifference, brilliance and stupidity, silence and speech, dependent always on the client's psychosocial needs and developmental vacuums. This is the prime message in "Casework with Ego-Fragmented Parents" and the papers on adolescents and group work with fathers.

Another dimension of the therapeutic process that has evolved in work with parents and children has been a growing respect for the client's resistance to change. Therapists now recognize that persuasion, suggestion, and even interpretation do not yield permanent changes in the client's life because the client, no matter how exact the therapist's statements, still seeks to maintain the status quo. The contemporary therapist tends to view the client's defenses or resistances as skin--they protect the person from injury. To pierce defenses and resistances prematurely is to produce blood. Therefore, the sensitive and skillful therapeutic surgeon reinforces and joins the client's defenses so that the client can give them up on his own, when, and only when, he is ready to do so by himself. This is the message of the Love and Mayer paper and the Nagelberg and Sternbach article. As the therapist supports and joins defenses, he is frequently experienced as an ally by the patient so that on his own he can climb the psychosocial ladder of development without prodding or seduction.

The insights emanating from the child guidance worker have been applied in child rearing, education, camping, and in many other areas of living. Principles which have been reviewed in the preceding paragraphs--joining resistances, supporting defenses, the corrective emotional experience, enactment of appropriate roles--are now being utilized by group workers, teachers, counsellors, etc. The papers on homesickness and "the age game" are included in this volume so that this contribution of child guidance may be partially illuminated.

In summary, child guidance has been drastically revised in theory and practice. Its unit of diagnostic and therapeutic attention has moved from the individual to the family, to the larger social system. Modalities and therapeutic arenas have been modified so that now group therapy, family therapy, institutional therapy, are in vogue. New theoretical perspectives are being utilized so that work with parents and children can be performed with more sensitivity, precision, and expediency. The client's defenses and resistances are more respected and the therapist has a richer repertoire of roles at his disposal to aid his client achieve a more enjoyable and mature level of psychosocial functioning. The following pages illuminate these developments.

Part I

Diagnosis and Treatment of the Child and Adolescent

2. Phobias in Children

by Hanna N. Colm

From The Psychoanalytic Review, vol. 46, no. 3, Fall 1959. Reprinted by permission. Dr. Colm originally noted: "Grateful acknowledgement is made to Claire Bloomberg and Sandra Kubat for assistance in the preparation of this paper."

Freud saw the experience of anxiety as part of the normal living of every human being. Its origin, he thought, lay in the fear of the infant lest he be deserted in his helplessness and immaturity without the protecting presence of his mother. In the course of maturing, the human being learns active ways of avoiding or minimizing his anxiety. If he fails to do this, but remains in the infantile state of passive helplessness, he becomes, according to Freud, neurotic.

To Freud's concept[1] of infantile anxiety as a danger faced alone without adequate protection from the parents, Melanie Klein[2] has added the concept that the danger which causes anxiety can also be some inner danger, such as the danger of one's own hostility and destructiveness, which in turn might cause the parents to desert or punish the child.

Following the lead of Harry Stack Sullivan on the interpersonal role which anxiety plays between people, I have observed that anxiety can arise in children not merely when they are threatened by an outer danger of desertion or punishment or by an inner danger of hostility which might lead to punishment, but more so in response to the anxieties of their parents, which spell to them, "I am not approved of." Mostly the anxieties of the mother are the ones to which the child responds with phobias merely because she is with the child so much more. Of course when the father is the parent from whom two-way feelings and anxieties come, he can also cause phobic reactions in the child. As there is virtually no published material on the relationship of phobic children to their parents, I would like to present for further research and comment my observations on children's reaction to parental anxiety, particularly where it leads to the development of phobic defenses. My conclusions are the result of my experience with a great many parents and children, seen both for analytic treatment and for short-term diagnostic consultation including Rorschach examination.

As I attempt to show in this paper, the mother's anxiety is felt by the child as an emotional desertion and if he is steadily exposed to it, this may become a cause of extreme and unbearable counter-anxiety in the child. A child can--and normally has to--accommodate himself to a small amount of anxiety in his mother, especially if he knows what his mother is anxious about and what she wants him to change. Feeling threatened in his security, he yields and changes his way of acting which seemed to have caused his mother's anxiety, and a healthy situation of learning results. When his mother's anxiety is too intense and too severe and persistent and the mother's defenses against it are too confusing to the child, the child will respond in a neurotic way.

There are different reactions on the part of the child to this threatening situation of severe, persistent anxiety. As I said before, a healthy reaction to anxiety in the mother can occur only if the anxiety is related to the living of the child, is occasional and then not severe: "I don't want you to touch this." Here the child learns from her anxiety and changes under her guidance, because he wishes to insure her good will and be comfortable again with her, and to keep her protection in future uncomfortable situations. This reaction does not need to be neurotic--all early learning and adjusting goes along these lines. But an unhealthy, neurotic, over-conforming reaction will necessarily develop when the anxiety of the mother is too intense and constant and rather unfocussed and general, often not related to the child's living at all, and when she tries to cope with it generally in her living via magic rules and controls. Wherever there seems to be an opportunity the child will compulsively comply with her defensive, magic ways of coping with her anxieties and fail to develop as a person on his own. The child's compulsive compliance with his mother may be aimed at controlling and avoiding the breakthrough of his own panic.

A second reaction might be an attempt to defy his mother as a different but also quite desperate means of winning control over her. Like compliance in a cooperative sense, defiance can also occur in all ages as a normal and healthy reaction, especially in adolescence, when defiance has its function in the struggle of the boy or girl for his own style of life.

Still another reaction might be either partial or complete withdrawal from his mother's anxieties. When the anxieties of the parent are so severe and diffuse that the parent cannot gain any control over them, or if he succeeds in keeping them almost completely out of awareness, in control, the young child is exposed to too much free-floating or intangible, unfocussed anxiety and he will withdraw completely. This is the background of the autistic child. The special type of also rather unfocussed anxiety that arises in parents when their conscious demands on their child are in conflict with their unconscious directions to him is a cause of partial withdrawal in children. In this situation the child is confused and can neither comply nor defy but takes refuge in misplacing his anxiety and hate reactions, which always represents withdrawal from the relatedness to his parent and from the situation which created his anxiety.

Phobias provide children, via misplacement and withdrawal, with one way of dealing with a panic experience. In phobias the child concentrates on one aspect or one symbolic substitute of his anxiety, which seems to give him freedom from generalized anxiety. Unlike the compulsively over-controlled child, whose behavior is still directed toward dealing with his parents, the phobic child no longer allows himself to be aware of the real conflict, which is always between him and his parents. Instead he withdraws and hides his conflict and his reaction to it by taking refuge in misplacing his fright and hate onto an object on which he can focus less anxiously.

In this article our questions are: In phobia, how

does the child's panic develop out of the situation in which he gets conflicting signals from his mother? How does his defense of concentrating on a part of the anxiety-creating situation, or on a symbolic substitute, usually work? What causes the selection of the specific object of his phobia?

As I said above, all phobias in children are dynamically caused by a very specifically disturbed relationship with the parents or other significant persons of their lives; the relationship of trust is either disturbed in a very specific way or was not allowed to develop. This happens because these significant persons' behavior toward the child is conditioned by their own underlying conflict between the conscious desire for him to obey or accept frustrations and the unconscious fostering of negative reactions. To the child this means that he constantly receives conflicted messages, which sends him into helplessness and panic.

The behavior of parents of phobic children usually falls into one of two types. Parents of each type, both the too-lenient, vacillating parents and the over-controlling parents, often have themselves had parents who were too rigidly severe or too lenient, or who disagreed between themselves in the handling of their children, leaving them to be buffeted about with no consistent standards of conduct along which to integrate their own behavior patterns, often causing in them a burden of unconscious antagonism which they have been unable to afford to express in their childhood.

In one case, unsureness about when and how to set limits easily, makes the parents anxious when the situation demands that they curb their child. "Love" means to them allowing the child to have what he wants when he wants it. They do not recognize that a child who feels secure and basically loved wants to follow his mother's lead and will yield in his unreasonable demands out of affection. They react to the child's difficulty in accepting frustrations in terms of their own unresolved anxieties about frustration. Such parents are driven by their conflicts into waiting "patiently" (actually anxiously) too long before taking action and falling then into an utterly helpless infantile rage.

In the other case, parents try to ward off helplessness by maintaining rigid control. They are on guard to keep their unconscious conflicts in check by severe rules and regulations on themselves and their children. Anxiety prevents them from spontaneously sizing up the situation as it arises; control serves to keep helplessness from awareness but often only barely hides their unconscious wish for the child to side with one or the other factor in their conflict. Caught in their conflict and narcissistically busy with themselves, they are unable to be guided by the child's needs in the situation; and the child senses not only that the parent is anxious and unsure but that conforming to rigid rules is on the conscious level of utmost importance to the reassurance of the parent. Unforeseen situations for which there are yet no rules cause anxiety and a child-like mistake or breach of regulations is also sensed by the child to be a cause of panic in his parents. It touches their inner unconscious conflict and may break through to their wish for rebellion, to which they secretly seduce their child.

In addition to the frequent similarities in the family backgrounds of parents of phobic children, the behavior patterns described, though often appearing nearly opposite, have common denominators. Another factor which is common is that in the homes of phobic children a great deal of talking on the adult side goes on and the talking does not correspond to what the parents really feel. Through talking they try desperately to feel at ease in setting limits, keeping at the same time their unconscious conflict out of awareness. But the child senses what goes on. The talking is a manifestation by which the child feels most keenly the discrepancy between his parents' conscious and unconscious wishes. For the parents, the talking is an attempt to reassure themselves and to produce a surface look of security and peace. But the talk is anxiety-ridden--compulsive--contradictory to what they unconsciously convey to the child and the child senses the intense, anxious unsureness and rebellion and resulting hostility of the parents, and is only further confused by their attempts to cover over and control through talking. For both parent groups the same factors are involved in the phobias of the children: the parents cannot themselves cope in a healthy way with situations that cause anxieties, nor can they help the child with his own anxieties, because they themselves are unaware of the fact that they unconsciously want something from the child that is contrary to what they consciously think they try to do. The child cannot trust the parents to help him as he needs to be helped but feels he has to join them in their defenses in order that they may be reassured. In many situations he even feels he has to act out what they unconsciously want him to do (and consciously don't want him to do). In both cases there is a terrible feeling of being alone when help should be forthcoming, especially when there is so much talk about love, rules, standards and security. Parents whose children react with phobias are using the child to live out their own unresolved childhood needs of rebellion and antagonism, utterly unable to see or follow the needs of the child. They do not find solutions which in terms of their present-day life meet both the child's and their own needs. In both types of parents with phobic children the vital factor is their unconscious inner conflict which the child senses and which causes unbearable confusion and helplessness in him, to which he reacts in panic and reliance in phobic defenses.

The root of the child's panic lies in the feeling: "I cannot trust my parents--they are conflicted themselves and unsure, helpless and not at all up to my immature impulses and demands." These children vaguely feel that their parents unconsciously seduce them into rebellion against accepting limits: "They let me take advantage of them--I can play on their problems and needs; they don't seem to discover when I am defying them and seem to foster my defiance. They take it for cuteness or playfulness, they let me manipulate them into anxious arguing and bribery and other helpless attempts to make me pretend to accept and even show phony enthusiasm for a necessary frustration, and suddenly snap out of patience into rage when I touch an unknown point, and I feel frightened. If they are not able to decide for me and help me over and through frustration, how can I feel supported and reassured? They seduce me to play out their hidden needs, not mine." Often a child feels additionally: "My parents are not together in their unresolved needs--I can often play off one against the other. How can I know when I have to take frustration, and that I can take it? How can I do this myself, when they are divided and so very uneasy about it?"

For the sake of clarity, I would like to point out here again that all human beings are more or less anxious, for many and various reasons. It is part of normal living. Many parents, when they become anxious, try to control and push down anxiety, sometimes to the point of over-control. The child of such parents will easily develop compulsive reactions, becoming himself over-controlling, eager to conform and even outdo what the parents demand, or he develops his own compulsive, magic attempts at rules. It is against a *specific* background of *conflicting anxieties* on the part of his parents that a child develops a phobia.

In the phobic child one of the most frightening experiences is the vagueness of anxiety due to conflicting inner demands in the parents; anxiety is there, where warmth should be. The development of phobias occurs always as a defense against the contradictory anxieties of the parents which the child feels as lack of concern. He feels left alone in the midst of vague, conflicting, surrounding anxiety and consequently full of hate and then guilt about his hate. The child takes refuge, in this most confusing and helpless situation, in partial withdrawal from the reality of the frightening situation; in place of the parents he hates and fears an object and thus manages to evade the most frightening interpersonal situation. With parents who are unaware of the contradictions between their conscious and unconscious drives, he misplaces the anxiety onto something that often pertains only symbolically to the real situation, of conflict between him and his parents; and the phobia contains strong factors of evasion and withdrawal from reality because of the discrepancy between what the child too strongly senses as his parents' conscious and unconscious demands. Still, the child does not withdraw entirely: he feels that the parents, though over-identified with him and over-reacting to him, yet are somehow busy with him, in some vague and distorted ways related to him. He retains his relatedness to them: his phobic anxieties serve to force their help to make them take clear-cut action so desperately needed by the child; it engages them on a different level of interaction, in which the child vaguely feels is hope for a more clear-cut, more constructive relationship. The compulsive child, because there are fewer unconscious and confusing seductions coming from his parents, can still hope to cope with their anxieties directly through controls such as the application of rigid rules or magic motions. In contrast to the phobic child's partial withdrawal and the compulsive child's more or less direct attempt to cope, the autistic child withdraws completely: he is overwhelmed by his parents' free-floating anxieties or by their preoccupation with controlling their intense anxieties that are completely out of awareness. He experiences their persistent anxiety and their attempt to control it as non-relatedness to him; and as a reaction to their lack of relatedness he does not respond to the outside world.

There are other factors that enter into the actual phobic experience. Usually, in his phobia, the child experiences a nearly infantile rage against the double frustration of his immature impulses as well as the frustration of not being helped. He feels forsaken and seduced, or anxiously confused with phony talk. He fears his own untamed impulses and their outbursts which he is powerless to control, while his mother with her two-way feeling and conflicts only shows an anxious, helpless, arguing approach to them, or an over-controlling approach which barely hides her helplessness as well as her unconscious seduction. He hates his frightened, confusing, seductive mother, who cannot accept him as an immature child and at the same time uses him for her own unconscious needs, thus not helping him gradually to give up his infantile wants--to yield as a gratification of their mutual affection.

This hate, which is engendered when the parents fail him again and again in his greatest need--the need for understanding help and control from outside himself--is a fearful and guilty hate, and is an important factor in phobias. Behind this hate reaction, which takes the form of extreme anxiety, is the feeling, "You don't help me, mother, and expect me to be able to handle a situation in which you, yourself, are helpless and anxious--I hate you." The hate factor in the phobic child is usually repressed because it is usually strong and therefore censored, as it is very threatening to a child to hate the persons on whom he feels he depends. The more the factor of hate toward the parent has to be pushed under, the more anxiously the phobia misplaces the expression of this hate onto more alarming symbols, thereby helping him to withdraw from the parents. For the clinician the phobic object usually gives some information about this process: it reveals in clear terms both how the child feels about his frightening impulses and his hate and how he tries to cope with what is to him an utterly confusing and alarming situation. Since his parents cannot be trusted to control him and the situation, he must get in control, and the phobic symbol is his means to this end. At the same time, his hate causes him to rage against himself in self-condemnation, and his phobia becomes partially self-punishment.[3]

Thus the real cause of the child's anxiety is always covered up by displacement onto something that he can try to control or avoid, but the displacement always contains symbolic reflections of the impulses which are frightening to the child and whose frustration he still hates, and of his inner rage toward his helpless and seductive parents, with the consequent need for self-punishment.

Specific phobias.

I would like to discuss the meaning of some of the phobias of children, as I have encountered them. Phobias of fire and fire engines invariably contain the experience of forbidden impulses and wishes with the child (often possessive and sexually colored wishes toward one parent) and the fear that the fire (the impulse) might get out of control. The character of diversion of impulse and hate onto the fire is obvious. What is really feared and hated here is the rage toward the parent who will not help him accept limits, but who unconsciously seduces him and allows him to go too far. Thus the terror "I might go up in flames" also serves as a severe form of self-punishment. Often, in this connection, the fear as well as the hope that his rage might be detected and punished may lead to a phobia of policemen. At the same time that the child fears detection, he is angry with the parent for not having detected his impulses, and helped him to resign them--give them up. Children often show phobias of fire-engines and ambulances, which do not, as one would expect, symbolize a source of help and comfort. On the contrary, they symbolize the fact that there is need for help (somebody's impulses did get out of control--mine could too) and the child fears that they will come too late, and only at the completed fact of outburst--just as his parents, who are never in time. At the same time, this violent fear serves as punishment--the more violent it is, the greater the crime. We can usually observe the child, in his forsakenness, gets his confusing and helpless parents into his control through his panic and achieves some degree of control of the situation.

In my experience, phobias of wild animals can usually be traced back to the impulse toward and the fear of the child's own destructiveness and its potential outburst, to which he feels secretly seduced by his parents. The animal in a way has a double face--fear and hate--where the child sees mirrored his own wild, uncontrolled wants and impulses--he wants to follow the seduction of his parents and fears it--and also his hate because his parents let him get out of control. Phobias of the dark reflect the same anxieties--fear of the child's own hidden and hostile impulses, projected on the world outside "there in the dark." His fear of the unknown, the dark, also expresses and avoids the vagueness of his parents' unconscious seduction which throws him into panic because neither he nor they can see it. Again often both fearing and wanting detection, he is afraid of some wild animal, such as a lion, which mother does not see because the dark hides everything. In reality, it is invariably the lion in himself which the child fears--his hostility--usually against one or both parents, who not only do not suspect the lion in him, but also unconsciously contribute to his scary inner situation, to which he can only react with rage. He uses his fear as self-punishment, and as a means of bringing his parents under an exasperating control.

I have only rarely seen claustrophobia in children, and then merely in forms of intense anxiety when doors were closed on them. In my experience, this also usually originates with anxieties about too few or too intense restrictions, again against a background of parents whose conscious directions were in conflict with their unconscious messages. Here, again, the dynamics of behavior are the same: the wish for limitlessness and the fear of it, the hate of the confusing, non-limiting parents and consequent need for self-punishment, and finally, control of the parents through the panic.

Phobic fears of dirt, brown paint, and the toilet usually arise in response to a mother who is on the surface, with her attempts to talk casually, consciously lackadaisical in toilet-training and helping the child toward cleanliness, though she still unconsciously demands a super-clean child; or to a mother who controls her anxiety and her own impulses about dirt by being very strict in her training while she unconsciously seduces him into rebellion against co-operating. Lenient mothers often do not themselves make these demands verbally on their children, but they are actually extremely anxious for them to live up to certain standards which they mention in the name of a teacher or the neighbors. Whether it be overt or covert, the important point in the situation is the underlying anxiety of the parents, which is apparent to the child no matter how "casual" the surface talk.

In these cases, the child is panicky about touching or using the toilet, or having any contact with dirt. With a lackadaisical mother, whose pretense he senses, he anxiously avoids a situation which calls for <u>his</u> managing and controlling--a thing he is hardly able to do, since the urge to mess is still too close to him. With a rigid mother, he feels her hidden anxiety and conflict about dirt. Unable to cope with her own unresolved conflict about infantile messiness she is unable to help him accept <u>some</u> dirt and <u>some</u> mistakes in his progress toward a socially accepted way of dealing with it. In both cases, he is actually afraid of his own enormous urge to be messy and indulgent, and anxious lest he act out his hostility by increasing his messiness. His panic serves as an outlet to his angry hate--through it he controls his mother and punishes himself. Phobias about <u>medicine, doctors, new foods</u> or <u>solid foods</u> also belong in this group. In these cases the child cannot comfortably take a new and hard step in any direction--new food, new medicine, an injection--because he cannot trust his mother to help him; this makes him hate her, and the vicious circle described above begins. Though she may try to hide her unsureness and apprehension under a cloak of casualness in the face of new and difficult experiences, the child senses her conflict and her unconscious identification with his immature side and is driven by his own feeling of forlornness into rage and hate and a complete inability to cope with the situation. When his rage and hate assume panic proportions and are displaced onto the actual food or medicine, we are again dealing with a fully developed phobia, which again contains a strong factor of self-punishment along with an overwhelming need to control the unsure mother.

One of the most widespread and crippling phobias is the phobia of <u>school,</u> on which a separate paper could be written. In my experience, school phobias are usually related to the child's anxiety about letting go of one or the other of his parents, more often his mother. In most cases, the child feels his mother's unconscious involvement with him, her need to keep him close and uniquely tied to herself for her own emotional satisfaction; like her child, she is unable to accept limits--she needs and demands a boundless relationship to him. His neurotic response to his mother's needs means that, with a part of him, the child indeed loves to be the special one--to have such power over her--but, at the same time, he is even more at the mercy of his hatred against being tied to her and kept away from his own life. He feels he is expected to serve the needs of his mother, overlooking his own, and the prospect of going off to school and leaving her evokes the familiar pattern: hate, resulting panic and the fear of giving up his substitute for love and trust--his power over her. His anxiety about holding onto mother and his need to control her as well as his anxiety about his hate is diverted from the over-all relationship and hidden in the concentration on his fear of school, the place where one would be able to go if the hateful and binding relationship did not exist. The self-punishment angle is obvious here--he will lose ground in his school work, and worse still, he will lose face with his peers.

At some time or other in the course of growing up, most children display some short-term phobic reactions. These occur as a momentary defense reaction, and are not to be confused with the actual day-to-day pattern of response which is the neurotically phobic child's reaction to the conflicting messages of the parents. But in my experience every real full-blown phobia, not merely temporary fear reaction, has a background of a parent-child relationship in which the parent is unconsciously conflicted about how he wants the child to accept limits and handle his impulses--his "I want what I want when I want it."

Still, I wish to stress that not all unconscious conflicts in parents produce phobic reactions. Children's procrastination or rebellion against authority and pressure or lack of authority and pressure, for instance, are often also an outcome of the conflict between parents' unconscious messages and conscious demands. "I hated being pushed as a child and I will not push my child"--and the parent withdraws from any help or guidance or pressure but unconsciously pushes the child because he has experienced it himself and knows no other way.

Phobia, then, is only one response of children to their parents' unconscious conflicts. Rebellion, procrastination or even complete withdrawal may be others. The type of reaction which children develop depends probably on the degree the child is threatened by the confusion in his parents and the degree of anxiety provoked. A completely withdrawing child seems to me basically a more anxious child than the child who withdraws only partially or who copes with the confusion by launching a rebellious or procrastinating power-contest which might bring the parent into a clearer position in relation to the child. One can also say that the different reactions of children to their parents' unresolved conflicts reflect to some degree the child's hopefulness or despair about the prospects of getting the parents into a more helpful interaction with him.

To summarize: All real phobias carry strong hate toward the parents who have unconsciously deserted the child or seduced him to their need. In addition, as the child is vaguely aware and non-acceptant of his hostility and anger toward the parents on whom he nevertheless depends, there is always an attendant factor of self-punishment in phobia. The phobia serves the purpose of localizing the vast anxiety in the face of his parents' self-centeredness and hatefulness by concentrating on an object, rather than on the disturbed relationship. With part of himself, the child tries to follow the conscious lead of his parents and control his immature, untamed impulses while, at the same time, the very fact that he is a child makes him easy prey to their unconscious seduction. In the interaction between parents and child, one might almost say that the phobia serves the function of controlling them to the point where they become alarmed, and thus are forced into some action toward helping him cope with a situation that is too difficult for him alone. The symptoms become alarming to the parents, they sense the child's anxiety and often even his hate, and are pushed into some angry action or become aware that they, themselves, need to seek help.

I have selected two cases which epitomize all the dynamic factors mentioned, factors which have presented themselves over and over in my work with phobic children.

Clinical examples.

Brenda is a girl of seven, the only child of elderly parents. She was brought to me because of her intolerable phobia of dogs, her consistent phobia of fire engines, and a recurrent phobia of lions, the latter dating from a visit to the zoo with her father.

Both parents had had deprived childhood experiences. Mrs. X had lost her mother when she was ten, at which age she was forced to assume the role of mother to a family of seven other children; Mr. X had lost his father when he was fourteen and carried the burden of earning a living for a family of six. In relation to Brenda, the parents seemed to react to their deprived childhood experiences in different ways. Mrs. X could never set limits for Brenda; she indulged all her baby demands, gave her whatever she wanted and allowed her to do as she wished. In my weekly work with her it became evident that underneath her identification with Brenda (" she should never have a frustrating mother"), Mrs. X was actually raging at the never-ceasing demands of the child, which she could neither face nor handle. On the surface, Mr. X was quite different--he demanded toughness and a nearly adult efficiency from Brenda. Beneath his high standards, however, was a very soft heart which actually sided unconsciously with Brenda's rebellion against growing up.

In appearance the child herself combined the tight face of a little old woman with a baby body--flabby flesh, round cheeks, short, fat baby fingers--and baby walk when she came for a psychological examination. She pussyfooted into my office and showed immediately that she was to have what she wanted. When I asked her where she wanted to sit, she chose first one place, then another, then went back to her original choice after all. When I then changed my approach and asked her to sit in a specified place for the examination she became more relaxed but became tense as she started the Rorschach. Her characteristic pattern clearly showed covered-over hostility, preoccupation with displaced anxiety objects (dogs, lions and fire), guilt about hidden hate (responses of "eyes looking at me"), and answers reflecting tendencies toward self-punishment.

My psychiatric work with this child revealed that her preoccupation with dogs was related to her anger towards her mother, who allowed her to have her way in all regards and unconsciously became more and more furious with her. In a number of pictures she showed me her envy of the neighbor's dog, toward whom her mother was openly furious for trespassing in the flower bed. That dog was the target of open and clear-cut feelings. The envy and anger which Brenda felt toward this dog (and actually toward her mother) were haunting her day and night and kept the child and her mother in an anxious involvement until Mrs. X would finally collapse and become openly furious at Brenda's demands in a guilty outburst, whereupon Brenda could then relax for a day or two, having received both direction and punishment from her mother.

It became clear in the treatment of this child that the fear of lions and fire engines was related to the parents' inability to set limits, particularly in regard to the father-child relationship, and to Brenda's angry guilt as she was constantly allowed to take advantage of them. Mrs. X frequently suggested that father and daughter visit the zoo, actually to have peace from the family tension herself, but with many verbal explanations that they needed a loving time alone. Behind his apparent demandingness, Mr. X was only too willing to have a loving time alone and to give his child the father experience he had never fully enjoyed. Though Brenda took advantage of this situation, she was actually torn between conflicting feelings: she wanted to be "daddy's girl" and to secretly trespass on her mother's relationship to her father, and at the same time she was furious that her mother allowed her to get into a "little love alone." In the zoo lions she had visited with her father she met the symbol of her fury about her mother's indulgent identification.

Since my office was located next to a firehouse and engines frequently passed by, I had an opportunity to witness Brenda's panic when this occurred. As frequently occurred with children in treatment, the sound of the sirens precipitated immediate, intense anxiety: "It has burst out--fire! It's too late, it has gotten out of control--help, help, help!" Brenda needed to rush out to the waiting room to reassure herself that her mother was still there and had not been burned up by the fire (her anger).

Treatment of this child and her parents lasted over two years, during which Brenda lost her phobias permanently; she has been symptom-free now for more than three years.

The second case is that of an 11-year-old boy and his parents which illustrates the family-relationship pattern which I have seen in a great number of cases as the underlying factor in school phobias.

David's parents described him as a very obedient boy who was somewhat uneasy socially. He had difficulty making friends, and tended to cling to home and especially to his mother. A frequent subject of their conversations was his difficulty in making friends, with David confiding his anxieties to her and she anxiously offering encouragement, mostly in the form of assurances that he certainly would soon make friends. It was unconsciously evident to the child how little his mother actually trusted that he would be able to make any healthy social adjustment. She greeted him daily with long inquiries about the friendships of the day. He came with long stories about his sad failures.

David's sister, four years older than he, was popular and outgoing. The mother, an only child herself, had been very close to this girl before David was born; he had learned how to draw the mother's attention away from his sister by worrying her. This he found easy to do, since the situation of being the mother of more than one child was a very anxious and conflicted one for her. She had grown up in an extremely indulgent and protected relationship to her own parents and knew no other way to relate to her children. After David's birth she tried hard to give both children this all-out, all-protecting love. Though she actually felt conflicted about her divided love, she began to talk extensively to David about equal love and devotion. This concept of "even" and "equal" love and fairness caused her endless anxiety, since she needed to be the all-fulfilling mother to both children, but did not know how to relate to them both on an "equal" footing. She was never able to say "no" to any request of David's without first deciding whether she had said "no" to his sister recently; her decision was made on this basis. When the situation was such that a clear-cut limitation was urgent she would ask David to himself make the necessary decision; he had to help her avoid the unbearable conflict. She would plead with him for hours, trying to convince him how happy he would be with the decision he was to make. But David knew only too well that he had to decide because his mother, despite her expressed views, was unable to reach a decision that involved limits.

In this way David had been persuaded to "want" to go to camp. In the course of his mother's repeated and anxious assurances that he would love it even though she would miss him and even though she felt uneasy about it, David, of course, became uneasy and at the last minute did not want to leave. His father, having already paid $200 for the camp, forced him to go, but on visiting day the counselor suggested taking David home, which they did. After this experience David spent the remainder of his vacation at home, worrying his mother about his newly arising fear of going back to school in the fall.

At this point David's parents brought him to me for treatment. It was difficult for him to leave his mother in the waiting room and he worried for weeks that she might be too hot there with only a fan instead of an air-conditioner. Even here he had to take care of his mother's problems. He was sure that she was miserable without him, and kept her worried with his constant checking on her comfort.

Slowly and gradually he began to look at the situation in which he and his mother found themselves. The first time he tried to break this pattern and extricate himself he went into a full-fledged panic. That day he drew a dog on a tight leash, led by a lady, with the caption underneath "Who is the slave?" In an effort to make the lady "lovelier" he erased her so many times that finally the paper was torn and the mother was nothing but a ragged, torn, ruined and "left-over" mother. He was furious at being put into the position of the dog on the leash of his mother's needs and used his phobia to make her the one who was on <u>his</u> leash. Actually, as his drawing, erasing, and re-drawing illustrated clearly, both were enslaved, and both were furious. David's guilt and need for self-punishment were clearly brought out in his phobia of school, the one place where this unsocial and intellectual boy could find satisfactions on his own. After the first year of treatment, concurrent with tutoring, David could go back to school. The parents still felt that the disappearance of the symptom was only a small part of what they wanted to work out in their family situation and treatment continued for over a year more.

Treatment procedures.

Thus we see that the central dynamic factors in children's phobic defenses are their reaction to persistent and intense parental conflicts and anxiety, anger at their failure to integrate impulses and hate for parents because of lack of help and guidance toward this integration, with resultant guilt and need for self-punishment. In treatment it is not usually necessary to demonstrate for the child his use of the magic of self-punishment. He no longer will need to "earn" reconciliation through this magic when he has experienced and learned to trust a relationship in which there are elements of anger and limits without loss of love, affection and relatedness. Likewise, his dependence on his defensive displacement--his phobia--will gradually become less as he experiences that flare-ups of hate and anger do not damage central and vital relatedness and as they therefore become less frightening and threatening to him.

This suggests that development of trust is a primary factor in the therapeutic relationship involving phobic children just as disturbance or non-development of trust is the cause of the phobic defense. It is my opinion that success in establishing relatedness and in treatment of these children can only come about when the therapist has an analytically oriented understanding of the dynamics of phobic reaction and defense. Concurrent analytic treatment of the parents also is especially essential since, as we have seen, phobic children are actually accommodating the unconscious neurotic needs of their parents. In non-analytic play therapy in which permissiveness plays the central healing factor and the therapist does not necessarily need to bring to the child's awareness the underlying dynamics, there is a danger of the child's becoming more and more anxious since conscious or unconscious permissiveness was one of the factors originally creating his conflict. Only some analytically oriented <u>understanding,</u> conveyed not merely through verbal interpretations but through an experience of relatedness with the therapist and his <u>reactions,</u> can bring into the child's central awareness how his phobic defenses have hidden his demandingness and hate of unsure parents and his attempts to control or take advantage of their conflicts. He must <u>ex</u>-

perience that only trust and yielding, and not the magic of manipulation or self-punishment, is the way out of the loneliness and helplessness of hate which he has condemned so painfully in his phobia.

In contrast to the relationship to his parents, the therapeutic relationship must be geared to the child's needs. The phobic child can begin to grow--to accept limits--only when clear-cut responses, geared to his needs and those of the situation, come to him from the therapist. Because of this, the therapist has to be alert to the child's sensitivity and reactions to the therapist's needs; he might otherwise soon find the child placating him. In the course of learning to accept limits, in such a relationship of trust, the child will learn to tolerate his hate reactions when he is frustrated, and to recognize that anger and hate about frustration can exist simultaneously with affection. Treatment must also make him aware of the conflict between his demandingness, with which his parents unconscisouly side, and his longing for their help to fit in peacefully, which they consciously demand. The parents too need help to discover the extent of their conflicts about limits and where they unconsciously seduce the child into rebellion and retaining his demandingness. The child must slowly experience that what he fears in his phobia is misplaced, that through his phobic defense he is keeping from awareness the threat of his anger, hate and guilt and with it punishes himself. In the relationship of trust anger and guilt become less threatening and frightening and guilt and self-punishment obsolete.

Limiting the child at first only where it is necessary to create a feeling of acceptance in him, he must nevertheless be led to experience the impact and extent of his demandingness and his simultaneous fears of the limitlessness of the situation which he creates. Therapist and child begin to see together how he wants more than mere tolerant acceptance and limitlessness--how he is actually demanding help in meeting his frustrations, provided only that the helper is tolerant and acceptant of the hatred which the frustrations engender. In treatment he experiences a person who is affectionate but who does not equate "love" with "allowing", who can set limits and make demands and still withstand the onslaught of the child's hate when limits are set without loss of affection and without disturbance in their central relatedness. As treatment progresses and trust deepens the child can be openly limited wherever necessary and the emphasis gradually shifts from the setting of limits to helping the child see his reactions to limits--hate and at the same time relief. It is important that therapist and child see together how he begins to hate at the moment when limits are set, and at the same time really wants more than tolerant limitlessness. The child must see that, feeling entitled to what he wants, the only way he knows to cope with a frustration or denial is to want more urgently and to hate and then become guilty about his hate. Gradually he realizes that he is longing for someone he can trust to stop him and help him curb his impulses, simultaneously helping him accept and integrate his frustration and anger. In treatment he must find this person if he is to integrate the frightening experience of his hate toward a parent on whom he is still dependent and someone who in addition can do this without losing affection for the child.

Now he is likely to begin to feel, more or less consciously, "I can trust this person; he is concerned with *me* and not merely wrapped up in his *own* anxieties and conflicts. He helps me accept limits without confusing me and without losing affection for me." Still, the therapist's affection may often be challenged or frustrated by the child's resistance or refusal to cooperate and open up, to relate. For example, the child's assumption that the analyst, like his parents, really wants him to have what he wants might well tease and irritate the therapist to the point of anger. Although as I said before, experiencing the reaction of the therapist is paramount in successful treatment of phobic children, sometimes even serving to establish central relatedness,[4] here it is of utmost importance that the therapist show his anger and irritation to the child openly and *not*, like the parents, hide his reaction in phony talking or anxious control. A play-therapy approach of permissiveness, as his parents' permissiveness and involvement with their own conflicts, spells to the child lack of relatedness and affection; it is equally likely to spell lack of approval. Just as the child must experience that his own anger at frustrations and limits is not fatal to central relatedness and affection, so he must experience that the anger which he provokes in the therapist is not fatal. As the child demanded limits and help in meeting frustrations, so is he likely now to demand an angry reaction from the therapist; if the therapist cannot trust himself to anger, how can the child be helped to integrate and tolerate his own anger? Here is the point where the child can be shown how his demands on his parents and his manipulation and attempts to control their anxieties created irritation and anger in them, at the same time that the therapist, in contrast to the parents, shows him affection but unwillingness to be pushed again and again into irritation and anger. Out of mutual trust and love he slowly learns how to give in to "you can't" and how to deal with the anxiety and anger such a yielding brings about.

Through the relationship of trust with the therapist the child has found a person who sets limits without becoming anxious, who helps the child accept his frustration at limits and who, should he become sometimes angry, does not hide his anxiety behind words or other concealing or controlling devices but finds his way back to a helpful, affectionate, adult relationship to the child. With this person he will play out the original situation of limitlessness which caused his hate, using dolls or puppets or drawings. He may also work it through in relation to the therapist in the transference situation.

The problem for the therapist is to be aware that the child does not face his hate in the original emotional situation.[5] He hates the therapist for different reasons than his parents at home, precisely because the therapist does not react as his parents do. In treatment, hate is provoked by setting limits, not by anxious, conflicted, concealing behavior; and the hate for the therapist is intermingled or followed by a sense of gratitude that the therapist takes the adult role. The very ambivalence of this feeling leads us closely enough to the originally traumatic situation and brings "hate," which the phobic child was too scared to face, into his awareness.

Whatever the vehicle, the therapist has to be careful to keep from the conscious awareness of small children the hate of their parents. The younger ones especially still need and desperately depend on the relationship to the parents, "good" or "bad" though they be. The therapist accepts his hate, also playing the original situation out with dolls or in transference, but does not fully allow the child, especially very young ones, consciously to recognize the feeling of hate toward his parents. Such conscious recognition would be unbearably anxious and threatening. With older children there might be a casual and accepting reference to the child's feeling for the parents--when the dolls "hate" each other or the child "hates" the therapist, the therapist might say, "Maybe you feel so mad at mommy (or daddy) too sometimes?" This would bring awareness that hate is involved in his sickness and that it need not be frightening. The most important healing experience is provided in the therapist's response to his unfocussed and misplaced hate: gradually he is able to experience trust in the helpfulness and reliability of the adult in setting limits and tolerating his hate reactions. As his parents, too, find help in resolving or integrating their conflicts, the child learns in treatment to live with, accept and integrate frustrations and anger. As these become less threatening and portentious of anxiety, guilt and the need for self-punishment, less misplaced in phobic defenses, they work themselves out and the phobia disappears.

Notes

1. Freud, S.: Analysis of a Phobia in a Five-Year-Old Boy (1909). Collected Papers, Vol. 3. London: Hogarth Press and The Institute of Psycho-Analysis, 1950.
2. Melanie Klein: The Psycho-Analysis of Children. London: Hogarth Press, 1949.
3. The compulsively over-compliant child fears his hate towards the inadequate mother so much that he prevents the expression of his hate completely. He often develops, besides compulsive symptoms, psychosomatic manifestations of his repressed hate and anger.
4. For further discussion of this point see author's article, "A Field-Theory Approach to Transference and its Particular Application to Children," Psychiatry, Vol. 18, No. 4, 1955.
5. For this reason, there is no actual transference in the Freudian sense.

3. Learning for Spite

by Jacob Kesten

From Psychoanalysis vol. 4, no. 1, Fall 1955. Reprinted by permission of The Psychoanalytic Review.

Increased understanding of ego development within the last decade has led to new ideas and methods of treating people with emotional disorders. This paper will concern itself with an account of the treatment of a ten year old boy who presented learning difficulties. Particular reference is made to understanding the unconscious ego of this boy and the use of one of the newer techniques in treatment.

Introductory Remarks.

We know that a child frequently reacts to an unfavorable environment with negative attitudes, such as resentment, anger, rage, revenge and hate. Because these attitudes are often unacceptable to the child's conscious ego as well as to his environment, they are repressed into the unconscious part of the ego. There, unbeknown to the child, they exert a destructive influence upon whatever the conscious and realistic portion of the ego constructively attempts to do. Much has been written about successful treatment of children by the standard proven methods of psychotherapy such as interpretation, abreaction, play therapy, suggestion, environmental changes, and the use of a good relationship. The therapeutic method described in this paper consists of the reflection of the unconscious negativistic portion of the ego by the therapist. The rationale for this technique is based upon the idea that the child can better deal with his own repressed oppositional negative attitudes when they are presented to him as an external adversary. It is hoped that this technique would enable the child to observe an enemy hitherto unseen, to study its strategy, to make self-preservative counter strategic moves, to understand and control it, to redirect it, and thus be enabled to pursue his conscious desire for psychic progress and social growth.

Background and Explanation of Symptom.

Patient, a ten year old boy, was retarded two years in reading ability despite an I.Q. of 135. He complained that disturbances of thinking and concentration were forces that interfered with his conscious desire to overcome his reading handicap. Unable to explain the reasons for his difficulty, he resorted to the explanation that was given to him by his parents, namely, that he was emotionally blocked and in need of a tutor who would employ some kind of psychological magic to rid him of this block.

A study of the family dynamics produced the following: The parents were emotionally unable to love the patient unless he brought them academic success. The patient was emotionally unable to comply, although he consciously wished this, unless his parents first gave him unconditional love. The more the parents pressured patient to be successful, the more devastating were his failures.

Dr. Nathan Ackerman in his paper, "Interpersonal Disturbances in the Family" states, "If we aspire to specificity in family therapy, we would hope, if possible, to reduce the definition of disturbance to a single formulation of the interaction pattern of the family, which encompasses within it the dynamics of intra-personality processes. To achieve such formulation, it seems necessary to view the functioning of individual personality in the context of the dynamics of family role."

Dynamically, patient identified his parents with his unconscious ego, and by defeating them, he defeated himself. This unconscious central theme which originated within the family found its way into the social sphere. Unbeknown to the patient, his mode of relating to parentlike figures may be formulated as follows: "The only pleasure that I get out of life is to find out what the teacher or any parent-like figure wants of me, then to defeat him in his purpose regardless of what is is, even though I too am crushed in the process."

Description of Technique.

In the first interview, patient initiated contact by an enthusiastic handshake. He spoke freely and easily without help; seemed outgoing, bright, and delightfully pleasant. He dwelled at some length upon his former tutors who were unable to help him because they were not "psychologically trained." The emotional overtones in connection with statements about his former tutors clearly indicated the patient's delight in their failures with him. A slight feeling of remorse accompanied his statement that both he and his parents felt badly about his reading difficulty. When asked how he thought he could best learn to read, he produced two books that he had brought with him and spoke in detail about the way in which his former tutor worked with him. When it was pointed out to him that the very method that he described had failed with him, he reacted to this with the statement that the injection of some kind of psychology would surely produce success. His parents had assured him of this. He pressured that work start immediately because time was being wasted by merely talking.

In the second interview, patient again brought the two books and again pressured that the job of tutoring begin without delay. He submitted to a series of brief reading tests with the understanding that a re-test would be done three months hence for the purpose of evaluating the treatment. The grading was done in his presence. He seemed pleased with the few correct responses, and groaned at his mistakes.

From the third session on, the therapist adopted a deliberate therapeutic attitude that conveyed to the patient that the therapist was not interested in helping him to read. The therapist employed stalling tactics by telling stories, engaging in discussions with the patient and encouraging him to draw, use clay or play. The patient perceived this and confronted the therapist with his diversionary tactics. It was discussed with the patient that the therapist had nothing to gain and everything to lose by helping the patient to read. The therapist realized that the patient was very bright and with the therapist using his magic psychology, the patient would learn to read ever too quickly and then the therapist would be out of a fee. The patient reacted to this with amazement. The therapist explained that money was very important in life and was amazed that the patient could not see this. The patient threatened to stop coming. The therapist stated that he had anticipated such a possibility and realized that he would have to take this chance because surely he would lose out if he tutored the patient. The patient tried a moral appeal, referring to the therapist's devotion to his work. The patient also threatened to expose the therapist to his parents. The therapist insisted that his desire for fees transcended all of the patient's arguments. The therapist recognized the patient's right to be angry, gave him a great deal of sympathy for the unfortunate position in which he found himself. However, the therapist did not wish to be a failure either and why could not the patient understand his point of view. The patient laughed and stated that the therapist was using psychology with him. He tested out his idea by reading aloud. Stumped by a word, he pressured for a correct response. The therapist yawned, looked out the window, and pretended not to hear. The patient jumped out of his chair, held the book close to the face of the therapist, pointed to the word in question, and prodded for an immediate response. The therapist volunteered a word obviously incorrect from both syllabic and phonetic aspects.

The patient's hope that the therapist was using psychology perished. In an angry outburst, the patient expressed disapproval of the therapist and praised his former tutors. The therapist was quite sympathetic with the patient's feelings, recognized them as completely justified, and told several stories of people who also found themselves in similar unfortunate situations.

The patient came regularly twice a week and was never late. He found himself caught in a web. He enjoyed the sessions; his feeling were recognized; he felt understood; received sympathy, enjoyed the relationship and the stories he heard; felt respected and accepted. He was not pressured to learn. In fact, pressure was placed upon failure. Whenever appropriate, the therapist (tongue in cheek) lectured him upon the dangers of reading, offering incredible examples. For instance, when patient mentioned a movie that he had seen, the therapist hoped it was a talking movie. Silent films required reading of lines and should he learn to read in a movie, the chances of reading elsewhere would be severely impaired. The therapist drew fake diagrams and eyesight tables to further this contention.

The patient argued that he did not receive notes from other children because they knew that he read poorly. The therapist spoke of the value of illiteracy, citing examples that notes are frequently intercepted by teachers who might humiliate him or grade him poorly in conduct. Moreover this might foster in patient sneaky character traits. The patient reacted to the therapist's remarks with mirth and laughter and took delight in discrediting the therapist's statements. At times the therapist expressed the hope that when the time for the re-test arrived, the therapist would have succeeded in keeping the patient a failure.

Subsequently the patient brought numerous test papers into the interviews showing that he was improving in reading. He was very confident that the re-test would show that he had improved. Moreover his teacher had complimented him upon his improvement. The therapist pretended to be defeated by these signs of success and attempted to learn the patient's secret plan. The patient would not reveal "*his*" magic psychology. Pretended attempts to trick him into revealing it were met with giggles.

The patient had been reading one book after each session from a list given to the parents. At home he asked his parents to help him and they eagerly complied. The impetus to read appeared motivated by spite and stemmed from the patient and not from parental pressure.

After three months had elapsed the patient was eager to be retested. He seemed to be living for this moment. The therapist expressed the hope that the patient would show no progress. The patient confidently announced that he *knew* that he had improved. The grading was again done in his presence. Each time a response was checked as correct, the therapist groaned and the patient clapped his hands. The patient had gained nine months in reading ability during the three months of treatment. The patient then announced triumphantly that he had won over the therapist. His long suppressed negative feelings rose to the surface, and for the first time he felt his true feelings. He expressed direct hostility in an angry outburst, called the therapist names, and vowed never to return again for a session. He could get by now without the therapist; could study by himself and he no longer had need for the therapist. He had continued coming in order to have this day of triumph.

Now there would be no future fees for the therapist.

It was at this point that the therapeutic plan was revealed to him. His negative suggestibility was clearly shown to him and how it was used for his advantage. He had been put in a position of defeating the therapist in only one way, that was by learning. The patient's reactions were dramatic. He burst forth with laughter, walked around the office shaking the chairs and table as if he wanted every piece of furniture to laugh with him. The patient was enabled to utilize his new insight toward further growth in treatment.

Conclusions.

Herein is described a plan of treatment, differentiated, to suit the personality of one child. An understanding of adaptive and intra-psychic factors were essential for this highly focussed therapy. The therapeutic attitude on the part of the therapist had psychic repercussions in this boy. For the first time in his life, he was with a person who did not pressure him to achieve. In fact, pressure seemed to be placed on failure. The challenge to defeat the therapist was invoked for the advantage of the patient. He seemingly defeated a parent-like figure, not to his detriment, but to his advantage. Since the therapist's behavior seemed designed for his own personal gain (interest only in fee), the patient was invited by example to think and behave for his own advantage. Hostile energy that had been used to defeat his parents by failure became redirected toward constructive goals. He became more interested in defeating the therapist by learning than in defeating his parents by not learning. There was less of a need to fight pathologically for unconditional acceptance. The patient had the therapist as a new model for identification.

This procedure may be attempted with patients whose learning difficulties stem from unconscious resentment, and present strong involuntary characterological negativism. Also this method is offered not as a demonstration but rather as a suggestion for further investigation of the structuring of a relationship for therapeutic gain.

4. Superego Manifestations in the Treatment of a Four-Year-Old Boy

by Herbert S. Strean

From The Psychoanalytic Review, vol. 55, no. 2, Summer 1968. Reprinted by permission.

This presentation evolves from both a theoretical and a therapeutic dilemma that I experienced in my casework and psychotherapeutic efforts in work with preschool youngsters. For a number of years I had difficulty in reconciling Freud's famous dictum, "the superego is the heir to the Oedipus complex," with clinical manifestations of two-and-a-half-, three-, and four-year-old youngsters who appeared very preoccupied with standards of "good" and "bad," "right" and "wrong," and "touch" and "see, don't touch." I often pondered the latent significance of these youngsters' remarks, wondering whether they were reflections of imitation and identification, "pre-superego" signs, or self-preservative ego manifestations.

Aside from their theoretical import, locating the essential derivation of exhortations like "see, don't touch," "see, don't break," would inevitably have to call forth differential treatment approaches. Particularly were the treatment implications crucial when working with adopted or foster children, where appropriate guidance to "significant others" in the child's environment could have an enormous impact on the malleable youngsters' development. A final concern which had both theoretical and treatment pertinence was a frequent observation, namely, that children whose over-all functioning seemed to be at a pre-Oedipal and sometimes a preverbal level nonetheless demonstrated what appeared to be clear cut superego manifestations. One could hypothesize here either a regression, fixation, or lack of maturation of many ego functions with the superego not participating in the regression, fixation, or lack of maturation or else, perhaps, something like a primary autonomous superego, developing not entirely out of Oedipal conflicts but somewhat independently.

The attempt here is to discuss some of these concerns as they unfolded while treating a four-year-old boy, Andy. Although our discussion will be focused almost exclusively on Andy's superego manifestations (or possible signs of superego), a brief description of Andy himself is in order. Andy came to my attention while I was a fellow in an advanced training program of a treatment center for preschool youngsters and their parents in New York City. Andy was a likeable and attractive looking four-year-old boy with brown eyes and hair, even features, and an infrequent but contagious smile. He was described by all who knew him as an intelligent boy but one who had suffered from early maternal deprivation. His ego was constantly bombarded by immature needs and requests. Though seeking for relationships, Andy was very distrustful of his environment. He seemed to be attempting to develop mechanisms to protect himself against early psychological injuries. While reaching out for gratification, he was carrying a heavy burden by himself and experimenting to find his own limits. There was in Andy a great deal of autoerotism: excessive masturbation, enuresis, nose picking; also, there was much hyperactivity with alternate displays of aggression, timidity and shyness. At times he seemed hampered by his fear of aggression and showed periodic withdrawal in his play. Andy was further described as narcissistic, very involved with himself, not having genuine object relationships but relationships designed for his own selfish purposes.

When I went first to Andy's record to learn what others had said about this child's superego, anticipating clarification of my own questions, what I found was unexpected. At the age of 3-11, Andy was described by a psychologist as "a child with a strong ego who has difficulty reconciling instinctual impulses with a precocious superego." He had, according to the report, internalized high standards and adult values of appropriate and inappropriate behavior and tried hard to conform to them.

My conclusion after reading the report was that a child with high standards who was preoccupied with "good" and "bad" at age 3-11 must be showing precursors of a powerful superego. However, when I read the intake conference on Andy, which was written also at the time he was 3-11, it was stated that he had many fears and was not spontaneous. Just as I was beginning to conclude that his spontaneity was hampered by an inhibiting, powerful superego, the report went on to say that though his spontaneity was hampered and Andy was concerned with "good" and "bad," these facts were not necessarily conclusive proof that strong precursors of superego existed. The fears and inhibitions could be on an ego level.

I next read several reports of teachers. There I saw repeated references to Andy's "I don't care" attitude, his hitting children without provocation and without apparent guilt. There was the implication by one teacher that "we might be dealing with a psychopath"--a child without a superego or at best a limited one.

My next step was to consult the literature. Freud, in his paper "On Narcissism,"[4] written in 1914, first speaks of an ego ideal which measures the individual's actual ego. "The ego ideal is constantly watching the real ego and measures it by that ideal. For that which prompted the person to form an ego ideal was the influence of parental criticism, conveyed to him by the medium of the voice, reinforced as time went on by those who trained and taught the child and by all the other persons of his environment--an indefinite host, too numerous to reckon." Here, we have the first mentioning, so far as I could determine, of a faculty in the mind designed to measure the ego's behavior--a censoring institution.

Freud again speaks of the superego in Group Psychology and the Analysis of the Ego,[6] in which he alludes to the leader of the group as representing the superego, and the members' identification with each other as identification of egos. However, his finer elaborations and discussions on the superego are found in The Ego and the Id[5] and in the New Introductory Lectures on Psychoanalysis.[7]

In The Ego and the Id Freud describes the ego growing out of the id, and the superego growing out of the ego. While he hints that there are superego manifestations before the onset of the Oedipal struggle, "the superego is considered an outcome of the sexual phase governed by the Oedipus complex." Freud states that the superego, which stands in contrast to the other constituents of the ego, is not only a deposit left by the earliest object choices of the id--it represents an energetic reaction formation against those choices. "You must not do such and such," says the superego.

While Freud later distinguishes between the superego and the ego ideal, seeing the former representing the more punitive admonitions and the ego ideal the more positive values, in The Ego and the Id he apparently uses the terms interchangeably and says: "The ego ideal has the task of effecting the repression of the Oedipus complex and to that revolutionary event owes its existence. The parents were perceived as the obstacle to realization of the Oedipus wishes, so the child's ego brought in a reinforcement to help in carrying out the repression by erecting this same obstacle within itself." The strength to do this was borrowed from the father (in the case of the boy) and so the superego retains the character of the father. Freud points out that the more intense the Oedipus complex and the more rapidly it succumbs to repression, the more exacting later on is the domination of the superego over the ego in the form of conscience or an unconscious sense of guilt.

The superego, then, is the outgrowth of two important factors, one of them biological and the other historical, namely, the lengthy duration in man of the helplessness belonging to childhood and "the fact of his Oedipus complex the repression of which we have shown to be connected with the interruption of libidinal development." The superego, according to Freud, is the expression of the most powerful impulses experienced by the libido in the id. By setting up the superego, the ego tries to master the Oedipal struggle but places itself in subjection to the id. Whereas the ego, as defined by Freud, is essentially the representative of the external world, the superego is the representative of the internal world, of the id.

In "The Anatomy of the Mental Personality" (Lecture XXXI in New Introductory Lectures)[7] Freud describes the superego most lucidly and sums up what has been said heretofore. The ego, he points out, is formed to a great extent out of identifications which take the place of cathexes on the part of the id which have been abandoned; the earliest of these identifications always fulfill a special office in the ego and stand apart from the rest of the ego in the form of a superego. The superego owes its special position to the fact that it was the first identification and one which took place while the ego was feeble, and it was the heir to the Oedipus complex and thus incorporated into the ego the most significant objects--the parents. Because the child's ego is weak and he is therefore compelled to obey his parents, so the ego later submits to the categorical imperative pronounced by its superego.

Ferenczi later extended some of Freud's formulations on the superego. Ferenczi[2] felt that what was described by the terms of "ideal," "ego ideal," and "superego" owed its origin to the deliberate suppression of real instinctual urges which had to be denied and repudiated, while the moral precepts and feelings imposed by education "are paraded with exaggerated assiduity." Although painful to students of ethics and theologians, Ferenczi felt that we could not avoid the conclusion that lying and morality are interconnected. "To the child everything seems good that tastes good; he has to learn to think and feel that a good many things that taste good are bad and to discover that the highest happiness and satisfaction lie in fulfilling precepts which involve difficult renunciations. In such circumstances it is not surprising--and our analyses demonstrate it beyond any possibility of doubt--that the two stages, that of original amorality and of subsequently acquired morality, are separated by a more or less long period of transition, in which all instinctual renunciation and all acceptance of unpleasure are distinctly associated with a feeling of untruth, i.e. hypocrisy."

Linked to superego formation according to Ferenczi are anal and urethral features. The anal and urethral identification with the parents builds up in the child's mind a physiological forerunner of the ego ideal or superego. "Not only in the sense that the child constantly compares his achievements in these directions with the capacities of his parents, but in that a severe sphincter morality is set up which can only be contravened at the cost of bitter self-reproaches and punishment by conscience. It is by no means improbable that this, as yet semiphysiological, morality forms the essential groundwork of later purely mental morality, just as the physiological act of smelling (before eating) is the prototype or forerunner of all higher intellectual capacities in which there is a postponement of instinctual gratifications (thoughts)."

Ferenczi spoke about the importance and the usefulness of ideals for the child, but also cautioned about the harmfulness of exaggerated ideals. "In America children are very disappointed when they hear that Washington never told a lie in his life. When one little American heard that Washington never lied, he asked, 'What was the matter with him?' I felt the same dejection when I learned at school that Epaminondas did not lie, even in joke."

Because we are interested in Andy's superego as it showed itself in a therapeutic encounter, I would like to underline several points regarding the superego that Freud, Ferenczi and others have developed, inasmuch as these points may aid us in determining Andy's superego manifestations.

1) Though the superego is the heir to the Oedipal struggle, there is the slight implication that there are forerunners and precursors.

2) The superego is the result of both parents' admonitions, although Freud stressed the role of the father much more.

3) The superego reveals itself independent of the external stimulus. If I take a nickel and give it back, I can give it back because of internal admonitions pronounced by my superego or, on the other hand, I can give it back because I may get caught. If I give it back because I fear I will be caught, this is an ego manifestation--self-preservation. As Freud says: if objective anxiety or fear is dominant, we cannot speak of conscience or superego.

4) Because the superego is the representative of the internal world and in tune with the id, as Freud has shown, the strength of the id impulse can make the superego powerful. The superego can reflect harshness even when the upbringing is gentle and kind. (Not all obsessive compulsives with corrupt superegos had punitive parents!)

5) If the superego formation is dependent on key

figures in the child's environment we should be able to see evidences of changing superego patterns in the changing therapeutic relationship, i.e. with the therapist often representing a superego figure.

6) The superego does not have to be cohesive--it may be rigid and punitive in one area of life and benign and friendly in another area.

The following are clinical examples of what I consider superego manifestations of Andy. Reasons will be offered for calling them superego manifestations. I shall deal only with the first two years of Andy's treatment, which covers a period up to the age of a little over five years, when according to theory, at least, the superego should not be consolidated.

When Andy first started treatment, he quickly became involved in water play and slowly reported his struggle with enuresis. While he pleasurefully filled the basin with water, he began to reveal rather intense guilt when the water spilled on the floor. He said, "It is not nice to have water on the floor," and felt quite obligated to clean it up. Still later when I made a connection between the water play and enuresis, Andy exclaimed, "A boy four-and-a-half should never pee-pee in his pants or in bed. That's for the younger kids like Petie" (his two-and-a-half-year-old brother). Even when I remarked about the id pleasure involved in enuresis, he replied: "Mr. Strean, if you are going to talk about pee-pee again, don't speak about it that way!"

During his second year of therapy Andy and I did not have many discussions on enuresis nor was there much water play. At one point towards the end of the second year, he said, however, "I told my father to wake me up at night so I won't pee-pee in bed. It's not nice."

Another theme which came up for much discussion and play during the first year of therapy was Andy's relationship with his brother, Peter. To describe the relationship, he took one puppet in his hand and gave me the other puppet, and the puppets engaged in a first fight. When, on several occasions, Andy succeeded in hurting my puppet and making it cry, he remorsefully said, "Little boy, I'm sorry I hurt you. Don't cry." When I tried to state his struggle, mentioning the joy of hurting but the uncomfortable feeling afterwards, Andy said more than once, "I like to hit but it is bad."

During the middle of his first year of treatment, when Andy was faced with the possibility of a tonsillectomy and eventually submitted to one, we saw many interesting reactions in which, I feel, the superego was operating. He made me be a little boy who was punished by receiving a tonsillectomy. In addition to this tonsillectomy, I was to be eaten by a mysterious ghost. The reason for all this punishment, according to Andy, was: "Little boy, you have watched your mommy and daddy while they are in bed. When I play with mommy's fire box, you should not look. Go to sleep."

Toward the end of the first year of treatment, when Andy and I discussed separation for the summer months, initially he denied his hurt, saying he did not care, and threatened to throw me down a toilet or sewer. He soon followed this up by saying, "Look, dooty-head, I was angry at you because I'll miss you. I'm sorry I said all that stuff. I meant it but I didn't mean it."

During the course of the second year of treatment we saw further manifestations of Andy's superego. In late September Andy's mother was rushed to the hospital with an undetermined diagnosis. Initially, he handled this with his characteristic response, "I don't care," and said that he hated his mother. He was furious with me when I remarked on the possible feelings of hurt in the situation. After various unsuccessful attempts to deny the hurt, he eventually stated that his family did not like him and he was going to run away with "Butch," his therapist. Though we succeeded in travelling many miles away from the home where the landlady was mean, never gave food, never smiled, was very selfish, and though we built a hut together far away from everything, we soon became haunted by a Landlady Ghost.

In Andy's dealings with the Landlady Ghost, which occupied much of the second year's therapy, his superego became vivid amidst constant fantasies of killing and being killed. "Ghost, people should get along nice. Don't you believe in friendship?" "Mr. Strean, tell the ghost that she should smile, be friendly, pay attention to us--that's the way people should get along!" Even though Andy killed the ghost and even though his ego expected the danger of retaliation because he left home, consistent too were constant ethical statements about fair play. "Ghost, I think you're mean because you are hungry. I 'll give you some custard; then you'll feed me, and we'll both be nice. That's the way people should live."

Andy on nearing the age of five became very much interested in standards of appropriate and inappropriate behavior. When talking about the pleasures of playing with feces, he stated quite knowingly, "Playing with b.m.'s is all right for little children. It's fun but a boy of my age should play with paste and sand." In thinking of the possibilities of marrying his therapist, he philosophized, "I'd like to marry you but there are laws against men getting married; I'll marry the girl who has her appointment next door, instead." On meeting the girl who had her appointment next door, Andy, like a true gentleman, ran to the door and held it open as she coyly made her exit.

Finally, examples of Andy's superego were witnessed in his changing relationship to the therapist. Though he always, although at times subtly, showed his desire for a relationship, he used the therapist in many ways. Initially, and for quite some time, he made impatient and gruff demands on the therapist: "Gimme the candy or I'll kill you, dootyhead, dope," sounding like a predelinquent psychopath. Later, his statements revealed quite a bit of ambivalence: "Look, Butch-chum, you're crazy, gimme the lollypops." Still later, "Look, Butch, dootyhead, you are a dope but I like you"; and still later when I appeared too curious about his love life with the girl who had the appointment next door, Andy exclaimed: "Look, Mr. Strean, why don't you stop working so hard. You give me candy, grapes, you help me with the ghost; you're too kind--relax and take a vacation. I like you but please don't be so nosy."

Why can we refer to the above remarks and behavior of Andy's as superego manifestations? First of all, they involve categorical imperatives: "People should be nice!" "A boy of four-and-a-half should not wet his bed!" "Fighting is bad." "A boy should not look at his parents while they are in bed." Secondly, these remarks are indepedent of any external stimulus. The therapist did not insist that

Andy control himself from wetting. If anything, he stood for the id pleasure. The same is true regarding Andy's aggression towards his brother; he did not appear afraid of retaliation as much as he showed his concern with the fact that "fighting is bad." Whether it be in terms of fighting, enuresis, peeping, Andy seems to have incorporated values of right and wrong by the age of five.

While it is not within the scope of this paper to discuss Andy's parents, it should be noted now that they appeared as gentle, over-permissive, indulgent and not harsh people. Perhaps because the strength of Andy's id impulses was great and perhaps because there was no consistent adult available, he had to carry the burden of erecting a strong superego by himself. Later in the therapy he asked the male figure to offer more controls. As mentioned earlier, he indicated that the therapist was too kind and his father should wake him up to go to the bathroom. In both instances he was seeking controls.

The fact is, as previously stated, if superego formation is dependent on key figures in the child's environment we should be able to see evidences of superego change in the changing transference relationship. It would appear that, as Andy grew less suspicious of the therapist and more trustful, he incorporated aspects of my superego. For example, I repeatedly asked him if killing was the only way to solve things; if yelling at me was necessary to make his demands known. He, in turn, asked later, "Ghost, don't you believe in friendship?" Or, "Ghost, I'm going to feed you, then we can be friends. That's the way people should be."

In Anna Freud's _The Ego and the Mechanisms of Defense,_[8] concerning the separation of psychic functions into the three systems, ego, superego and id, she points out that these systems are clearly and sharply delimited only when they are in _conflict_ with one another. When an instinctual derivative arising in the id is acceptable to both ego and superego and is gratified by the individual in behavior or fantasy without arousing any inner opposition, it is not possible to say when the ego's defenses are opposed to the id impulse nor can one draw a sharp line between id and ego.

As Brenner[1] says in "The Concept of the Superego," the same description can be given of the relationship between ego and superego. If the two are in harmony, a sharp differentiation between them is impossible. In such cases it is often fruitless to ask and impossible to answer the question, "How much of what is going on is ego and how much is superego?" Such a question can usually be answered best when there is a degree of opposition between the two systems.

It would appear that the clinical material in Andy's case showed this opposition: there was the desire to urinate indiscriminately but we saw that wish opposed by Andy's critical self-observation, with definite standards of behavior. This was equally true regarding the play with puppets where we saw him hampered in carrying out his aggression because his moral standards inhibited him.

In analyzing the clinical examples I have given, we can, with some assurance, say that there are evidences of superego. What is perhaps most interesting is that here we have a boy with many pre-Oedipal difficulties, and many of his productions hint at life at a preverbal and pre-Oedipal level. Despite the fact that in the period described he was far from having worked through problems on pre-Oedipal and Oedipal levels of development, we have not only seen precursors of superego development, but many evidences of true superego. And when I refer to superego here, I mean a consolidated superego with aspirations, ideals, standards of fair play, ethics, morals, etc. This raises a most serious question. Does the superego form only as a result of working out the Oedipal conflict, as Freud seems to imply? Is it only the heir to the Oedipus? When Andy was 3-11 he was already preoccupied with "good" and "bad," and this preoccupation in therapy did not diminish, despite the abundance of his productions on pre-Oedipal levels of development.

If all the examples I have given of Andy's superego are really superego examples, it would appear that Freud's definition of the superego is too rigid, and the superego does not owe its origin solely to the set of conflicts activated by the Oedipal situation. As Freud expressed it, the superego is the heir of the Oedipus complex. If that is correct, from what we have seen of Andy, his superego, a kind which

Freud would call an Oedipal superego, began to reign quite early and powerfully.

Freud mentioned that the superego does not have to be cohesive. Perhaps Andy's superego offered different admonitions in a one-to-one relationship than it did in a group situation. One wonders if a therapist does not provide a different type of superego figure from teachers and if, for this reason, the therapist witnessed less of Andy's provocative, aggressive, seemingly superegoless behavior.

In summary, then, I would say that Andy was a boy who showed a characterological reaction to maternal deprivation. His ego was bombarded with immature requests and he was forced to carry the burden alone. Carrying the burden alone could conceivably lead to the development of a powerful superego, which I believe Andy had. Although far from successfully graduating from the phallic period and resolving his Oedipal struggle, nevertheless he consistently manifested a true superego in his therapy.

The implication here for therapy with adults is obvious. If there is a true superego before the resolution of the Oedipus, do we not find it incumbent on ourselves to relate to pre-Oedipal material with the realization that our patient is far from a naive child being exploited but "a smart kid" who in many ways "knows right from wrong." With the patient's knowledge of right from wrong on our side, the therapeutic task with many individuals may be not so much for the therapist to enact the role of "benevolent superego" (as is so frequently advocated) in order to reduce guilt, but to face the patient with his unrealistic pre-Oedipal fantasies which he inappropriately wants gratified, yet realizes simultaneously are "not right."

Notes

1. Brenner, C. _An Elementary Textbook of Psychoanalysis._ New York: International Universities Press, 1955.

2. Ferenczi, S. _The Problems and Methods of Psychoanalysis,_ Vol. 3. New York: Basic Books, 1955.

3. Freud, A. _The Ego and the Mechanisms of Defense._ New York: International Universities Press, 1946.

4. Freud, S. On Narcissism (1914). Collected Papers, Vol. 4. London: Hogarth Press, 1950.

5. __________. The Ego and the Id. London: Hogarth Press, 1923.

6. __________. Group Psychology and the Analysis of the Ego. New York: Liveright, 1922.

7. __________. New Introductory Lectures on Psychoanalysis. New York: Norton, 1933.

5. The Use of the Patient as Consultant

by Herbert S. Strean

From *Psychoanalysis and the Psychoanalytic Review*, vol. 46, no. 2, Summer 1959. Reprinted by permission of *The Psychoanalytic Review.*

While psychoanalysis, as a field of research and study, has always concerned itself with its own growth and has sought new replies to unanswered queries, it would appear that we are now witnessing a different phenomenon. Part of the very web of psychoanalytic treatment, with its emphasis on interpretive intervention, is currently under serious scrutiny.

What is precipitating this trend? Are cultural changes, which create new and different symptoms and character problems, bringing a new and different patient to the therapist's office?[10] Is psychoanalysis emerging from its latency period and feeling revived impulses to create?[6] Perhaps--but it is not the purpose of this paper to examine either the causes or the apparent modifications in the psychoanalytic community. That changes are occurring is quite clear.

One could cite numerous examples in current publications, all suggesting a shift of therapeutic attention to new themes and a unique assumption of a therapeutic role. Instead of interpreting pathological aspects of the patients' maneuvers, various authors have described successful attempts at role playing, mirroring the patients' distortions, joining their resistances, and supporting their defenses.[1, 4, 5, 8, 9]

The writer, a young student of psychoanalysis and psychotherapy, gradually grew apprehensive and confused as he was exposed to the current contributions suggesting modifications of traditional therapeutic technique. As he heard and read differing treatment procedures from respected supervisors, consultants, and authors, each new prescription for treatment became increasingly difficult to master. Like most students who struggle for a logical orientation to psychoanalysis, the writer spent many hours attempting to solve the dilemma. One of the ideas that evolved was a wish to see to what extent a patient could prescribe his own treatment and what results could be achieved through this procedure.

It is the purpose of this paper to describe, through case illustrations, the writer's experience in this therapeutic endeavor.

Case I--Joe M.:

Joe M., a fourteen-year-old boy, was referred to a child guidance clinic by school officials. He had failed several subjects, could not read, was very withdrawn, and participated in virtually no extra-curricular activities. His persistent negativism and social isolation were apparent in all of his relationships. He wanted "nothin' from nobody."

Prior to referral to the clinic, Joe had been involved with several therapists, but was able to defeat all of them. In each instance he withdrew from treatment and could not be persuaded to return.

It is quite clear why the patient intrigued the present writer. At a time when the therapist was struggling with psychoanalytic theory, treatment suggestions, and his role as a therapist, he could easily empathize with the patient's anger at and disillusionment with the authority, his defenses against the anger, a provocative negativism, a need to withdraw from the mainstream of life, and a fear of internal and external change.

Therefore, Joe was told in the first interview that he intrigued the therapist and the latter wanted to keep him in treatment. However, the therapist recognized with Joe that he had successfully defeated everybody in the past and it was a safe bet that the same thing would occur again. The patient was asked by the therapist, "What should I do?"

Joe responded, "I can tell that you are the same as the other guys and I'm not coming!" and remained silent for fifteen minutes. When the therapist found the silence unbearable, he told Joe that he reminded him of Gandhi, the Indian leader. Possibly he could teach the therapist techniques of passive resistance? After several statements by Joe showing continuing strong resistance and several anxious comments by the therapist that he wanted Joe to come so that he could learn Gandhian techniques, Joe told the therapist that he talked too much. When the therapist conceded that his patient was probably correct, Joe stated that he might try for a little while to teach the therapist to be silent. If he were silent, Joe might consider another visit to the clinic. However, the patient insisted, "You have to promise to say nothing; I'll be the boss around here." At that, the first consultation terminated. Directions: "Be inactive. Let the patient direct the process."

Several interviews passed uneventfully. Joe, instead of talking and teaching, remained silent. The therapist and patient merely looked at each other with no exchange except, "Hello" and "Goodbye." In the middle of the sixth session, Joe broke the silence and exclaimed, "I'm quitting; I don't like it. Nothing is happening. You are no better than the other guys." Here, the therapist replied that he must be doing something wrong. He asked Joe where he was erring and what could he do to make treatment worthwhile for Joe.

Joe told the therapist that he did not wish to demonstrate his techniques of passive resistance any longer. "I'm not getting anything out of it," he remarked. Though the therapist felt that he himself was getting something out of it, he wondered out loud what he should do now. Joe merely returned to his silence and doodled with a pen. He devised electrical circuits and fantasied how he would burn down the clinic. He cursed the therapist and the building in monosyllables, yet made it clear that he had some skill in electricity. When the therapist wondered if Joe could teach him something about electricity, Joe got up, walked out of the interview and stated dryly, "You've got a lot to learn. I'll think about coming back and showing you."

Joe did return for two silent sessions, but without encouragement soon delighted in showing the therapist several electrical plans. Electricity became the sole mode of communication for several months, with Joe as teacher and the therapist as pupil. However, again Joe's ever-present negativism asserted itself. He told the therapist that he was "tired of being the big shot" and that it was about time that something be done for Joe, himself. The therapist asked Joe what he thought could be done. The patient renewed his hostile barrages and stated that the clinic was the same as school, "plain awful." The only difference between school and the clinic was that at the clinic he could dabble in electricity. The therapist remarked, "You want me to do something. You like electricity. Maybe I can find you an electrical school." To this Joe replied, "There is no such thing; you could not do anything about it." Again the therapist asked, "What should I do?" He was advised "not to get so excited, do less talking and give with more action." At this point the therapist "gave with more action" and tried to find an electrical school.

Though it took weeks to find the appropriate school, Joe was extremely tolerant of the therapist's slowness. "Take your time, it's not that important," he frequently remarked. Eventually, Joe entered a vocational school and specialized in electricity. As he spoke with enthusiasm of his electrical pursuits and an occasional relationship he developed at the school, he finally confessed that he was learning how to read quite well.

As he learned how to read and attained other academic and social successes, Joe suggested that "the case be closed." He wrote in his own handwriting, "A Closing Summary on Mr. Strean" in which he both criticized and praised the therapist, giving a colorful picture of the treatment process.

The therapeutic encounter with Joe may be discussed from two focal points: namely, the impact of the relationship on Joe and the effect on the therapist. From Joe's point of view, he gained from the relationship and as time went on, he involved himself more in "treatment." Perhaps the main reason for his increased involvement was because there was no treatment to resist. The therapist was the patient, the learner, and the passive recipient of Joe's teachings. Furthermore, Joe's withdrawal was supported--he was compared favorably with a famous Indian leader. As the therapist disrobed his professional cloak, Joe was able to loosen some of his pathological defenses. When the therapist demonstrated that he could take from Joe, Joe began to think of asking for something from the therapist. As he saw that the therapist appeared relatively unthreatened as a student, Joe gave evidence of interest in school and in reading. In brief, Joe slowly identified with the therapist and became more of a human being.

For the therapist, the relationship had enormous meaning. By identifying with Joe, he received vicarious pleasure in knocking authorities. The patient's refusal to read and participate in school was similar to the therapist's condemnation of supervision, consultation and the literature. As Joe dabbled with electricity, the therapist enjoyed dabbling with what appeared to him as therapeutic dynamite. As the relationship between Joe and himself deepened, paramount, of course, for the therapist was a strong identification with Joe's emerging social interests. As the patient became interested in school, an illuminating insight dawned on the therapist.

The use of the patient as a consultant was, in reality, a combination and synthesis of all that the writer was consciously fighting. Working with Joe was really an attempt to "Treat an Untreatable Case."[9] It contained aspects of "Paradigmatic Psychotherapy";[1] the patient was being "mirrored" and the therapist was "role playing." An attempt was being made at "Healthy Insulation in the Withdrawn Child."[5] Certain "Irrational Trends in Contemporary Psychotherapy"[7] were being considered and unconscious stabs were being made at "Sector Analysis."[2] As the patient's negative therapeutic reaction was being dissolved, so, too, was the therapist's negative reaction to supervision. As Joe could take from the therapist and attend school, the therapist could return to his supervisors and give and take with them.

The validity of a hypothesis can, of course, only be confirmed with substantial empirical data. The following two cases, illustrating the use of the patient as a consultant, occurred after the experience with Joe. Here the writer, less narcissistically involved, applied further the above hypothesis.

Case II--Mr. L.:

Mr. L., a father of forty-five years, did not seek therapeutic help directly. Unknown to him at first, and later against his wishes, his wife applied to the clinic for guidance in relation to their only son, Morton. Twelve years old, Morton was a neurotic child. He had fears of the dark, strong feelings of inferiority, could not tolerate competition or aggression, was extremely passive and overly compliant.

Mrs. L. and Morton were involved in treatment for more than six months when the going got too rough for Mr. L. He objected to Morton's developing aggression and found it necessary to contact Morton's therapist. On the telephone Mr. L. explained, "I am coming down to bawl you out. You don't know what you are doing!"

Mr. L. arrived ten minutes late for his appointment. On entering the office, he took the therapist's seat and stated: "I am going to tell you a thing or two." He remarked that he knew all about this "social work stuff" and wanted to tell the worker that "there are many things wrong with the way social workers run their business." The therapist told Mr. L. that he was eager to learn about his mistakes.

Mr. L. vented a great deal of anger. He declared that Morton had to be dealt with very firmly or else "he would not be kept in line." He further remarked that "permissiveness is a lot of hokum and nobody should be molly-coddled. That's what you do to my son!" With encouragement from the therapist, Mr. L. offered several techniques on how young boys should be treated.

At the end of the first interview, the therapist told Mr. L. that he appreciated this consultation and had been very much enlightened. He invited Mr. L. back to the clinic for another consultation.

Mr. L. arrived on time for the second interview a week later. He proceeded to villify and condemn the therapist, clinic, and the profession once more. He suggested to the therapist that he "get out of the field and learn how to make money." The therapist responded, saying, "Maybe that's a good idea!"

In succeeding interviews, though with less rancor, Mr. L. continued to give advice on the treatment of people in general and the approach to Morton in particular. The therapist took notes very eagerly.

By the sixth session, Mr. L., much more subdued, told the therapist that he could have his seat back. He thanked him for "taking all of my advice and guff," stating that a big change had come over Morton. "I started to listen to his point of view like you did to me and it works like magic." Mr. L. followed this with a request to join a Fathers Guidance Group which the writer was leading at the time. "Maybe," concluded Mr. L., "I can learn from and teach the other fathers."

Using the patient as a consultant in Case II helped to initially involve Mr. L. in a relationship. His aggression was accepted and his ideas were considered important. Unconsciously, Mr. L. was recapitulating with the therapist what Morton was doing at his stage of treatment--acting out hostility toward the parental figure. As the therapist demonstrated a method of dealing with Mr. L.'s demands, convictions, and fantasies, Morton eventually became the recipient of a new mode of parental handling. As the therapist tried to appear unthreatened by Mr. L's barrages, Mr. L. endeavored to emulate this behavior with Morton. Mr. L. observed that the therapist was seeking advice, learning and sitting in the patient's chair; eventually he could do likewise.

While Case II manifests certain similarities to Case I in that problems of negativism, hostility toward the authority, fears of external and internal change are present in both instances, there are differences to be considered. Mr. L. was used as a consultant solely to involve him in a relationship. After he relinquished some of his defensive maneuvers, he asked for treatment. It is questionable whether he should be asked to serve as a consultant any further. Perhaps he is now ready to be approached through the medium of classical interpretive intervention.

After the writer's encounter with Mr. L. he realized more fully that the use of the patient as a consultant has to be used discriminately. With many patients, perhaps this technique can be used only at the beginning of treatment or at certain other crucial phases, rather than throughout the life of a case. As the patient reveals a different set of resistances, the technique of therapy must be modified.

Recently the writer has had the opportunity to serve as Intake Worker in a child guidance clinic. He has observed that numerous individuals, although they apply for therapy, are quite ambivalent about help. Their apprehension may be masked by anger and they are ready to challenge the interviewer and destroy future therapeutic possibilities. This is particularly true in the following case, where the patient did not seek help voluntarily.

Case III--Mrs. J.:

Mrs. J., an attractive woman in her early forties, was referred to the clinic by the court. Her fourteen-year-old son was found masturbating in the lavatory of a subway station. Arrested by the police, he was brought to court, put on probation, and ordered to seek psychiatric treatment.

On the telephone, Mrs. J. gave little indication of the problem. She did not mention that she was being referred by the court but instead bellowed, "My boy is going crazy. He is perverted. He may rape somebody any minute. He is deranged. I need help immediately." When the worker tried to explore what was crazy about the boy, Mrs. J. insisted that she could not commit herself on the telephone and needed to discuss her problem in a face-to-face interview. Although the worker tried to elicit more facts, he was unsuccessful.

Despite Mrs. J's pleas for help, when she arrived for her interview she blurted out, before being seated, "I don't belong here. I'm here against my will. The judge sent me here because they think my son is crazy. He is not. Do you think he's crazy?"

Trying to place the interviewer in the role of a judge, Mrs. J. castigated courts, the subway system, and psychiatry. Feeling discriminated against, she "had it in" for everybody. The worker, not wishing to be a judge, stated that he certainly was not capable of knowing her son's degree of health. He also told her that he realized that she did not want to be in the clinic. What should he do?

Mrs. J., although continuing to ventilate intense rage, gradually mellowed. She confessed that she felt embarrassed in talking about her son's arrest and the complications attending it. She begged the interviewer to write a letter to the court giving "my son a clean bill of health." However, when the worker stated that maybe he should follow Mrs. J's advice, and asked what he should write, Mrs. J. broke into tears. "I don't know what to say. I'm really very confused. It is hard to handle an adolescent boy. I have sexual problems with my husband. I need help myself. My boy needs help but I need it more. Could you treat both of us?" Mrs. J. went on to complete a series of intake interviews and eventually began therapy for herself and arranged treatment for her son.

What is interesting to note about this case is the contrast between Mrs. J's statements on the telephone with her initial remarks in the office. When she called, the worker attempted to explore the facts. This made him appear like a judge or lawyer and probably helped Mrs. J. strengthen her resistances. It may partially explain her strong negative reaction during the first few minutes of her face to face interview. However, when the worker refused to play the role of judge, abdicated his authority, and asked Mrs. J. for advice, the latter told her story.

Cast III demonstrates how the use of the patient as a consultant can help him over the difficult therapeutic hurdles of an initial interview. The first interview is often termed a "consultation"; if the therapist can assume the role of a consultee, he enables the patient, through identification, to experience the interview situation as less threatening.

Perhaps implicit in the use of the patient as consultant are the basic and generic concepts of psychotherapy. In the final analysis, the writer sees this therapeutic tool as embodying not only recent contributions to psychotherapy, but concepts taught to every beginning psychotherapist.

Among the more generic concepts inherent in the approach is that treatment cannot be forced upon another person. "Domination or paternalism, seldom, if ever, bring about effective results. Do not play providence and do not take the problem away from people; just assist them to mobilize their own capacities and to keep active as far as possible in their own behalf."[11]

Inherent in the application of the patient as consultant is the realization that therapists "shall not impose upon the client their own goals or standards of behavior, their own solutions and morals, but shall concede the person's right to be himself and make his own decisions and plans."[3]

As indicated, the intrapsychic process that took place in the writer while testing the methodology herein described, helped him to accept with more ease his role as a student and therapist. The use of the patient as consultant, if paraphrased, should read, "You teach me; I am ready to learn."

Notes

1. Coleman, M. L. and B. Nelson: Paradigmatic Psychotherapy in Borderline Treatment, Psychoanalysis, Vol. 5, No. 3, 1957. p. 28-44.

2. Deutsch, F. and W. Murphy: The Clinical Interview. Vol. II. New York: International Universities Press, Inc., 1956.

3. Hamilton, G.: Theory and Practice of Social Case-Work. New York: Columbia University Press, 1940, p. 6.

4. Nagelberg, L. and H. Spotnitz: Initial Steps in the Analytic Therapy of Schizophrenia in Children. The Quarterly Journal of Child Behavior, Vol. IV, No. 1, January, 1952, p. 57-65.

5. ______________ and Y. Feldman: The Attempt At Healthy Insulation in the Withdrawn Child. The American Journal of Orthopsychiatry, Vol. XXIII, No. 2, April, 1953, p. 238-252.

6. Nelson, B., ed.: Psychoanalysis and the Future, New York: National Psychological Association for Psychoanalysis, Inc., 1957.

7. Schwartz, E. and A. Wolf; Irrational Trends in Contemporary Psychotherapy: Cultural Correlates. Psychoanalysis and the Psychoanalytic Review, Vol. 45, Nos. 1 and 2, 1958, p. 65-82.

8. Spotnitz, H., L. Nagelberg, and Y. Feldman: Ego Reinforcement in the Schizophrenic Child. The American Journal of Orthopsychiatry, Vol. XXVI, No. 1, January, 1956, p. 146-164.

9. Sternbach, O. and L. Nagelberg: On the Patient-Therapist Relationship in Some 'Untreatable Cases'. Psychoanalysis, Vol. 5, No. 3, 1957. p. 63-70.

10. Wheelis, A.: The Quest for Identity. New York: W. W. Norton & Co., Inc., 1958, p. 17.

11. Young, P.: Social Treatment in Probation and Delinquency. New York: International Universities Press, Inc., 1937, p. 316.

6. Psychotherapy with Adolescent Girls In a Court Clinic

by Murray H. Sherman

From The Journal of Genetic Psychology, 1958, 92. Reprinted by permission.

Psychotherapy with adolescents in a court clinic involves many problems of technique which differ considerably from ordinary procedures with self-sustaining adults. Girls who come to our attention have been brought to court by their parents because of acute discord at home. Parental complaints include such disciplinary problems as late hours, promiscuity (often an unfounded accusation), and general disrespect. Most often it is the mother who brings her teen age daughter to court. In these cases the father is either ineffectual or else there is a total absence of a father in the home. The court then becomes a substitute to the mother for the weak or absent father.

The mother's own motivations for bringing her child to court have many unconscious meanings. Almost always we find that she has provoked her daughter's "wildness" by grossly inconsistent handling. The mother will repeatedly tell the girl what she should not do until she does it. Then both of them become overwhelmed by guilt, jealousy, and anxiety. The court is seen as a means for restoring some sort of equilibrium and both punishing and condoning all wrong doing.

Despite these many neurotic motivations of the parents, it has been generally necessary to treat the girls themselves with some hope of promoting a stable family situation. The girls' attitude towards attendance at the Clinic is almost always overtly hostile and negativistic to begin with. These negativistic feelings often conceal an underlying need to be forced into attendance, and the entire relationship to the Clinic is conceived of in terms of a sadomasochistic retribution for forbidden behavior. Even after a long period of friendly and cooperative behavior the girl may insist that she is going to see us only because she is being forced to do so.

Treatment techniques vary according to individual needs, but some common procedures have developed which seem helpful in many cases. Most frequently it is worthwhile to focus upon the immediate surface problems which have brought the girl to court. Usually she has been placed on probation and is overtly resentful of this fact. I may begin therapy by telling the girl that our aim is not to take sides either with the family or with the court, but instead to help her get off probation by clearing up whatever situation brought her to court in the first place. An approach of this kind will usually release a flood of accusations directed largely against her mother, although in many cases the father is made a substitute target because of intense fear of the mother. The cathartic effect of this release provides some ameliorative effect of its own, and it may then become possible to focus upon problems in school or on the job. It is rare that our girls have made a satisfactory adjustment in either area.

Very soon evidence of transference becomes apparent. This transference has all the elements of intensity and instability that is characteristic of the adolescent period. The girl may ask for a mild favor or concession on the part of the therapist. The loan of carfare money or changing the time of an appointment may serve her the opportunity for finding out whether the therapist is really on her side. It is often helpful to accede to these requests and to maintain the positive transference without any interpretation.

It has also been found useful to limit the intensity of the transference by giving the girl a minimal amount of appropriate personal information about the therapist, when this question arises in treatment. For example, if I am taking a vacation, I may tell the girl where I am going and a little bit about the place. This kind of information has the effect of limiting to some extent the romantic fantasies which most adolescent girls tend to build up about a relatively unstructured relationship. This limiting of transference also reduces the patient's guilt and anxiety regarding Clinic attendance and thus permits closer attention to other reality problems. In so far as the therapist can give structure and reality meaning to the therapeutic relationship, he tends to minimize the projection (i.e., transference) of unconscious erotic feelings by the patient.

If some progress is achieved by these techniques it may then become possible to help the girl to adjust to some parental demands. The lowered intensity of the general home situation has by this time resolved some of the more blatant stresses. The girl is frequently told that she must recognize the fact that her parents do support her and are legally entitled to govern her behavior until she becomes of age and is able to support herself. If a favorable relationship with the therapist has been achieved, there is usually an acceptance of these remarks.

Our techniques are in general oriented toward assuming a stable parental role toward the girl. It has been found most helpful to take the part of a firm but kindly adult, who is benevolent but consistently authoritative in attitude. After parental relationships have improved to some extent the girl may begin to bring up material which would lead to unconscious motivations and this area is approached slowly. With some girls the anxiety aroused by these unconscious problems provokes a flight into mental health, and therapy may well be terminated at this point. The girls who continue treatment in order to probe unconscious problems are usually those with rather well developed character neuroses or borderline schizophrenics, and these girls often present prominent sado-masochistic behavior involving promiscuity or prostitution. Some case material may further illustrate these problems.

Louise R. came to the attention of the court when she was 16 years old. She was brought to court because of continually staying out until two to four A.M., occasionally running away for as much as a week at a time and for using vile language toward her mother. Mrs. R. was a jealous, moralistic woman who was married for the third time, her first two husbands having died. Louise's father had died when she was four months old. There were no other siblings. Mrs. R. said that Louise was completely out of hand and she accused her daughter of promiscuous behavior and of striking her.

Upon referral to the Clinic, Louise appeared as a

tall, attractive, maturely developed girl (IQ of 101) who spoke in a frank and open way but was resentful both toward her parents and the court. She was particularly bitter toward her stepfather who, she felt, had no right to tell her what to do. She insisted that she had never been promiscuous and had never really struck her mother except in partial self-defense. Mrs. R. had continually annoyed Louise by prying into her dates with boys, insisting that Louise was little better than a whore and at the same time warning her against sexual indulgence. Louise had already left school and held several jobs as a bus girl. She said that she usually was insulted by her bosses who made sexual advances or spoke harshly to her, and she usually left her job within a matter of weeks.

Louise was seen in therapy once a week for 16 months. For about the first eight to 10 months the storms at home continued but with gradually diminishing intensity and frequency. One of the major bones of contention was Louise's boy friend, Marty, who had been sent to a reform school for theft. Mrs. R. was extremely upset at the fact that Louise maintained contact with Marty and that she intended to marry him when he was released. The therapist kept showing Louise how these arguments at home served to keep her on probation and in trouble with the court.

It gradually became apparent that Louise's temper outbursts had started about the time that her mother married for the third time. It was also about this time that she started to go with Marty. Louise then described her mother's attachment to another man with whom she had gone prior to her present marriage. This man had found it necessary to take a long trip and had asked Mrs. R. to wait for him. However, Mrs. R. was an extremely jealous person and continually accused him of having left her for other women. She finally could wait no longer and married Mr. R. Nevertheless, Louise felt that her mother was still sorry that she did not marry the man for whom she had been waiting.

It became obvious that Louise's waiting for Marty represented an unconscious desire to show her mother that she could do what her mother had failed to do, i.e., wait for a man whom she loved. However, as this parallel came closer to the surface, Louise's behavior improved in a striking way. Under our direct guidance and support she had undertaken and completed a secretarial course and she now got an office job with a large commercial firm. She now shied away from any discussion involving her mother, and spoke of how extremely happy she was with her work. She was making far more money than she ever had and found that she was able to accept many of her parents' unreasonable demands upon her. She was content to spend most of her time at home or with girl friends and now got along quite well with her mother and even with her stepfather. Mrs. R. became overly solicitous and protective, and in fact insisted upon kissing Louise each day before she left for work. Although many personality problems remained, Louise was poorly motivated for continuing treatment, and it was felt that our major goals had been accomplished.

To illustrate some of the problems and techniques of treating a more disturbed girl we present the case of Marjorie T. Marjorie was a moderately attractive Negro girl of 18 (IQ of 116) who came to the attention of the court because of a first offense in prostitution. She was well motivated for treatment and related to the therapist in both an intellectual and seductive way.

Marjorie described herself as having always been a decidedly seclusive girl who had done well in school but made no friends. She said that she liked to observe life objectively and that she hoped to become a writer. Marjorie was seen at the Clinic once a week for a period of eight months, and it took almost this amount of time to get a clear picture of her life behavior. At first she was difficult to follow in her associations and showed some pressure of speech. She dwelt at some length on early childhood memories and showed a striking lack of infantile amnesia.

Marjorie was the third of four children; her siblings were all boys. She had not been staying at home when arrested but had told her parents that she was married to George W., the man with whom she was living. Marjorie explained this relationship in a blatantly illogical way. She said that while visiting George one night she had become so sick that she could not go home and so spent the night with him. The next day when she left for home and got near the house, she felt that she could never explain the situation to her parents and so went back to live with him. After this incident George became abusive and jealous toward her. He did not allow her to get clothes from home even though she had only one dress to wear and frequently he did not let her leave the house.

Her relationship with George had been a markedly ambivalent and sadomasochistic one. She loved him as she had never loved anyone else, but at the same time she hated him because of the way he treated her. She was passive and compliant in her overt behavior and accepted his beatings. However, she planned to kill him and put some sleeping pills in his coffee. Then she changed her mind, drank the coffee herself, but did not suffer any ill effect. Marjorie prostituted herself at George's insistence in order to provide him with money for drugs, since he was both an addict and seller of narcotics. George then became involved with the law and was sent to prison. Marjorie decided to prostitute herself one more time in order to get money to live by herself and then get a job. It was, of course, on this occasion that she was arrested.

Marjorie's parents had come from a highly moralistic background and expected her to be totally chaste. Her mother had continually pointed out the women in the neighborhood who had a shady reputation and warned her to avoid this road to degradation. Mr. T. was very strict and demanding in his attitudes and had beaten Marjorie savagely when she was a child.

The patient's early memories included her fears of being poisoned and of being abandoned by her mother. She also recalled that as a child she had thought that she was a boy and that she had a penis which was as yet flat and undeveloped.

Marjorie's course in treatment was an extremely stormy and uneven one. It was soon recognized that prostitution had served Marjorie as a means of getting even with both of her parents. The therapist pointed out that prostitution had also gotten Marjorie into a great deal of trouble with the law and had actually hurt her more than her parents.

After the patient had ventilated many of her feelings

and early memories we began to focus more stringently upon her job situation. It then became clear that Marjorie had definite paranoid ideas regarding her employers and felt that they knew of her prostitution and would call the police or take sexual advantage of her. This material was dealt with largely in terms of telling Marjorie that, although there might be some basis of fact in what she said, it would be necessary for her to continue working and to try to overlook some of these things.

A particularly acute episode of this kind occurred at the start of a menstrual period and Marjorie came to the office in a highly agitated and hyperactive state. She said that her boss had accused her of being seductive toward him and this had made her tremendously resentful, offended, and agitated (her own provocative role was clear in what she said but this, of course, was unrecognized by her). Marjorie had also been quite seductive toward me, but had denied any thoughts of this kind. She now said that she had not had time to eat, was hungry and offered some candy she had brought. I accepted the candy without interpretation and dealt with the job episode as illustrating the fact that she would have to disregard any advances her boss made. The many interrelationships among Marjorie's menstruation, the candy offered me, the drugs supplied to George, and her early fears of being poisoned were not dealt with at all.

After this session Marjorie improved steadily in her vocational adjustment and was able to get the kind of job she wanted on her own initiative. However, she tended to take jobs which would be temporary and worked considerably below her own level of capability. Her social life remained rather barren, but she was able to capitalize on some intellectual interests. Subsequent follow-up indicated that Marjorie formed relationships with men who liked to gamble or drink. She was not interested in getting married and recognized the fact that she could relate only to men who seemed deviant or mildly asocial in some way.

In evaluating the factors influencing Marjorie's return from prostitution to a more satisfactory and socially acceptable work adjustment, it is felt that the therapeutic technique resembles that of Louise despite the wide differences in clinical symptoms. In both instances the patient's improvement was due in part to ventilation of hostility and other feelings towards the parents and in part represented an escape from insight regarding more incentuous material. Louise improved in her behavior when her own jealousy toward her mother became implicit in what she was saying. Marjorie improved when her own provocative role became implicit both on the job and in the transference. Both the jealousy and provocative behavior were accepted without interpretation. In Louise's case, acceptance was indicated by complimenting her on her vocational adjustment without pointing to its defensive aspect. In Marjorie's case, acceptance was signified by eating her candy without interpretation of its symbolic meaning.

These techniques are oriented toward limited goals which have been dictated both by practical administrative needs and also by the nature of the patients themselves. It may be argued that "deeper" insights might have provided a more beneficial effect than the limited interpretations given. I doubt that this would be true for the majority of girls seen at our Clinic, but it must be admitted that the personality of the therapist is a crucial element in work of this kind. Our point of view is that we are serving the community as well as the girl herself and that the needs of all are best met by promoting relatively stable relationships in the home and at work.

Essentially our technique involves the use of an unconscious incestuous conflict with the parent-therapist as a stimulus for initiating the adolescent's growth away from her mother. It will be recognized that this defensive flight from the parents is also prominent in the normal adolescent who does not come for psychotherapy. In this sense we are deliberately providing our patients with a significant relationship which is necessary to an adult development.

Summary

This report describes psychotherapeutic techniques which have been found useful for dealing with adolescent girls in a court clinic. It has been found helpful deliberately to assume the role of a firm but benevolent parental figure and to limit the intensity of the transference. These girls are able to improve their life situations by developing some minimal insights into day-to-day problems and ventilating their feelings toward their family and toward the court. It has also been found that these patients can improve their adjustment by developing behavior which is a defense against understanding deeper unconscious problems. In general, our technique involves a cathartic working through of surface problems and the direct encouragement of subsequent defense formations.

7. Difficulties Met in the Treatment of Adolescents

by Herbert S. Strean

From Psychoanalysis and the Psychoanalytic Review, vol. 48, no. 3, Fall 1961. Reprinted by permission of The Psychoanalytic Review.

Tradition holds that radical changes take place in the developing human organism as it emerges from childhood into maturity. This transitional phase, known as "adolescence" is therefore regarded as one of crucial importance. Like all transitions, it is marked by instabilities and by shifting back and forth from old to new behavior and from old to new attitudes. Most investigators have agreed that adolescence is a period of "storm and stress" and heightened emotionality.[15]

Anna Freud has lucidly described the adolescent's plight in The Ego and the Mechanisms of Defense.[10] She particularly calls attention to the resurgence and intensity of pregenital and oedipal impulses which sharply conflict with the ego's refusal to resort to the well-known solutions of infancy and latency. This leaves the young person more difficult to reach, control and teach.

Anyone who has lived or worked with adolescents has noted their many struggles on all levels of development. Their oral conflicts appear in hoarding food or abstaining from it, as well as in peculiar choices of food mixtures. Anal sadistic activities are frequently observed--"foul" language and disregard of, or excessive preoccupation with, clothes and cleanliness. Phallic and oedipal interests are embodied in the images of heroes on the movie and television screens.[2]

Peter Blos has stated, "The pivotal problem of adolescence is the problem of object relations."[3] The polarity of active and passive aims re-emerges and the earliest passive dependency on the mother possesses an alluring attraction for the adolescent of both sexes. The stronger this passive need, the more archaic becomes the defense against it by rebellious fantasies and actions often resembling infantile range. The adolescent becomes increasingly self-conscious about physical contact with the parent lest any infantile dependency needs assert themselves. As he withdraws cathexis from his parents, we inevitably see a remarkably narcissistic individual with a heavy concentration on his personal processes (beliefs, interests, opinions, likes and dislikes).

The adolescent's unstable body image frequently manifests itself in attitudes of shifting interests, mood swings, and fantasies not always clearly delineated from reality. This is expressed in turn, in waves of ecstacy which fade into discouragement, boredom, and discontent. Adolescents are ". . .excessively egoistic . . .and yet at no time in later life are they capable of so much self-sacrifice and devotion. They form the most passionate love relations only to break them off as abruptly as they began them. On the one hand they throw themselves enthusiastically into the life of the community and, on the other, they have an overpowering longing for solitude. They oscillate between blind submission to some self-chosen leader and defiant rebellion against any and every authority."[10]

Eissler has emphasized that adolescence "may end in suicide if the resistances to and the fear of impulses and fantasies concerning heterosexual or substitute gratifications are so strong that the ego cannot cope with the new demands upon the psychic apparatus."[7] It is because the ego is working so hard coping with so many demands that some analysts do not undertake treatment of adolescents on the ground that psychoanalysis cannot be useful for this age group.

Because of his powerful narcissism and frequent lack of relatedness, his mood shifts, intense negativism, impeded functioning of ego faculties and fragility of defenses, the adolescent has often reminded the clinician of an adult schizophrenic. Many writers have noted that the psychic processes occurring during puberty have similarities to those occurring during psychosis.[12, 9, 2] Furthermore, the controversy regarding the adolescent's therapeutic inaccessibility is indeed somewhat reminiscent of the perplexities encountered in the treatment of the narcissistic neuroses. Like the borderline or psychotic, the adolescent frequently seeks to establish distance between himself and the therapist by engaging in antisocial behavior or by asocial withdrawal.[33] As Fairbairn has described the borderline schizophrenic, "His overevaluation of mental contents and close association of giving with self revelation cause him to perceive the therapist as an intruder who will shake a tenuous economic balance."[8] So, too, with the adolescent, the advent of the therapist is usually seen as an anxiety-provoking situation. He rarely comes for treatment of his own accord, but is brought by some outside agent, like the parent, school or police. If the therapist is perceived as a source of gratification, he represents a threat to the ego's attempt to protect his infantilism. If the therapist is seen as a representative of society's social demands, he then threatens the containment of aggressive impulses.[33]

While engaged in the treatment of adolescents this writer has frequently experienced in his therapeutic encounters similar feelings and reactions induced by borderlines and schizophrenics. Work with adolescents seems to demand a similar vigilance for attitudes of irritation, hurt narcissism, or unresolved anxieties in oneself. Like the borderline, the adolescent is more skeptical of all types of "would be" and "as if" attitudes and frequently reacts unfavorably to friendly support.[26, 6]

Just as in the treatment of schizophrenia "the analyst becomes increasingly aware of the need for more subtle intervention than is possible through classical interpretation,"[25] therapy with many adolescents requires techniques which can be employed in the analysis of resistances, defenses, and fantasies that are not amenable to classical interpretive intervention.

During the past several years numerous authors have suggested new stratagems that have been used effectively with borderline schizophrenic patients and appear to have much relevance in the treatment of the disturbed adolescent. (5, 7, 11, 16-18, 20-25, 28, 29)

The treatment technique that has most profoundly influenced this writer in his work with adolescent patients has been the use of paradigmatic psychotherapy designed primarily for the borderline schizophrenic patient. The rationale and procedures of this form of therapy have been discussed in several papers.[4, 5, 25, 30]

Paradigmatic techniques are employed in the analysis of resistances and defenses of those patients whose irrational egos cannot tolerate classical interpretive intervention. For patients whose integrative capacity is limited and who need help in identifying primarily what they feel rather than why they feel, the therapist strategically selects certain types of roles and offers himself as a model for introjection and identification so that ego growth can be promoted more effectively.[5] Mirroring the patient's distortions, joining his resistances, participating in his fantasies, reduplicating introjected images are among the many stratagems employed in paradigmatic psychotherapy.[25, 5]

The remaining portion of this paper describes various paradigmatic approaches found appropriate to the treatment of certain resistive adolescents who could not respond to classical therapeutic intervention. The cases selected are not meant to encompass the rich diversity of adolescent patients and their various responses to the therapeutic encounter, but attempt to highlight a few situations where the prospect of therapy appeared particularly upsetting to the young patient and the continuation of it was very much in jeopardy.

Part II

Most adolescents do not come for treatment on their own accord but are frequently ordered to see a therapist by their parents, school, or some authoritative person or agency in the community. The complexity of this situation and its psychological implications often oompound existing resistances to treatment.

> Steve, age 15, was picked up by police authorities several times after he had been found truanting from school. He hated school and all that it implied--"horrible teachers, dumb kids and dull subjects. Why the heck should I go there? There are better things to do!"

> When Steve met his therapist, he very quickly transferred to him all the qualities of a strict school disciplinarian. "What the heck do I want to do with you? There's nothing wrong with my head, Doc! I bet you work for the school, anyway, and you only want to get me back there. You are a head shrinker and you know it."
>
> On being told by the therapist that he had no interest in getting him back to school, "because that would be a pretty dull job for a head doctor. I had better things to do anyway" Steve responded, "So what the heck do you want with me?" The therapist stated, "Not a darn thing!" Steve tried to cover up an anxious smile by saying, "You're pretty wacky aren't you? Are you some kind of fairy?" The therapist responded, "Maybe I am. Sometimes it is hard for me to understand myself." To this Steve managed a mild giggle and exclaimed, "You must have been an interesting jerk in your day." He speculated that the therapist was a criminal "let loose from a booby hatch" and was never caught. He wondered if the therapist had ever gone to college. "You mean with horrible professors and stupid college students?" the therapist queried.
>
> Steve went on to say that this conversation was "O.K." but he didn't think he'd want to visit the therapist again. Then after a long pause he said very quietly that maybe he'd come back in three weeks if he had nothing else to do. "Three weeks," the therapist exclaimed, "why not six months?" The remainder of the interview consisted of an attempt on Steve's part to convince the therapist that maybe another "bull session" would be in order.

While the events of this one initial interview are rather dramatic and the movement rapid, the interview tends to demonstrate an adolescent's struggle in meeting a therapist for the first time and suggests some means of helping him cope with the burdensome situation.

When Steve arrived at the therapist's office he was ready to meet somebody who would be exactly like a police officer. He attempted immediately to knock the therapist's authority and induce the therapist to respond with anger and perhaps punish him. However, when the therapist told Steve that he was not interested in sending the "wayward youth" back to school, he was able to accomplish two things. First, the role that was ascribed to the therapist had to be questioned by Steve. Secondly, Steve could become a little interested in the therapist who appeared like Steve himself, a rebellious deceiver.

It seems imperative in the establishment of contact with a highly narcissistic adolescent that the therapist resemble some aspect of the patient.[3] This technical maneuver of becoming part of the adolescent's highly cathected self-image has been developed by Aichorn in his book, Wayward Youth,[1] and elaborated by Hoffer in his article, "Deceiving the Deceiver,"[16] Steve, after perceiving the therapist's behavior as similar to his own, could become a little intrigued with somebody who seemed to resemble himself.

During adolescence, when the ego is working overtime in coping with internal stimuli, the young person often resorts to a primitive mechanism, namely, projection. Steve felt the need to ascribe many of his own intolerable thoughts to the therapist. "You are a fairy, you are a jerk, you are a criminal." Rather than interpret the adolescent's distortions, it may be more helpful to the patient if the therapist listens attentively to the accusations and temporarily takes them on his own ego. As the therapist appears relatively non-defensive about the qualities ascribed to him, the youth is grateful to the adult for accepting these noxious elements and slowly questions how dangerous they really are.

Many patients, in general and adolescents in particular, have their own preconveived notions as to the way the therapy should be conducted. This defensive maneuver wards off any therapeutic intervention which may disrupt the patient's tenuous psychological balance. The paradigmatic psychotherapist often utilizes the concept of self-dosing,[25, 30] thereby joining the patient's resistance, and invites him to recommend procedures for the therapist to follow.

> Jack, age 17, had successfully defeated two therapists. The product of two overly-intellectualized

> parents, he rebelled against the idea of accepting his therapist's interpretations as he did his parents' overpromotion of intellectual accomplishments and school teachers' directives. Jack had his own ideas of how things should be done.
>
> When Jack's third therapist actively enlisted his direction on how the therapy should be conducted, Jack gave many prescriptions. "First of all, I am not interested in your opinions. You should just listen. I have a lot to say. Then I have my own ideas about dreams. Not that Freudian stuff. Also, I'm not calling you by your real name. I'm calling you String Bean. You look like one."
>
> The therapist complied with his patient's instructions and for many hours maintained his silence, interrupted only once or twice during an hour with a "Right, Mr. Jack." Jack, for six months twice a week, made the therapy room a lecture hall. He presented his ideas on philosophy, sociology, psychoanalysis, sex and religion, without a challenge or question from the therapist. Finally, with strong anger, he bellowed in his fifteenth session, "Why are you so lazy? Can't you get off your stupid rump and help me? Aren't you tired of listening to me by now?" When the therapist responded calmly and stated, "I'm only obeying orders," Jack spent several hours castigating the therapist for listening to a person younger than himself, urged him to get to work, and offered many items for a realistic analytic agenda.

Jack had a strong need to assume an active role in the therapy and to have the therapist become the passive recipient of what he, Jack, had experienced in the past. He behaved with the therapist like his mother and father did with him, lecturing, advising, and not permitting any intrusion. The therapist not only permitted Jack to receive the gratification his parents did not allow but also demonstrated by his behavior that intellectualized speeches do not necessarily have to ruffle the listener.

Of course, the therapist did not agree with every recommendation that Jack offered. He merely refrained from interpreting Jack's behavior and did not challenge him.

Then, and only then, could the patient feel sufficiently protected and relinquish his defensive maneuvers by himself.

Because of his intense negativism, when the therapist does not initiate psychoanalysis the adolescent, after going through a period of active testing, often asks for treatment.[17] As he sees the adult appear relatively unthreatened by the patient's advice and counsel, the young person may venture to seek help for himself. To quote Hoffer: "Aichorn's main device seems to be arousing surprise without causing fear, establishing strength without threatening, pretending to attract without promising anything. He utilizes any weakness the adolescent may show, outdoing the impostor's tricks in a cleverly conducted fantasies a deux.[15]

Many young people, defending themselves from unbearable ideas and impulses, develop an obsessive interest in a sport figure or movie hero and may use countless therapeutic hours just discussing the personage from every point of view. In the treatment situation this may be used to deflect any arousal of transference fantasies.

> Twelve-year-old Sally came to therapy with many phobias. She was afraid of the dark, the elevator, animals and burglars. Not consciously pained by these phobias and receiving much secondary gain from them, she used her therapeutic hours to discuss Marlon Brando. Everything--his eyes, ears, speech, clothes, hair, family--was Sally's concern. The therapist listened attentively and in appreciation, but periodically would refer to Shirley Temple. He told Sally of the clothes the actress wore and discussed with enthusiasm the movies where she was the leading actress. Sally appreciated the therapist's admiration of Shirley Temple and the therapist showed keen interest in Mr. Brando. Hardly anything was discussed but Brando and Temple.
>
> During Sally's seventy-fourth hour she remarked, "Do you always have to talk about Shirley Temple?" The therapist innocently queried, "Why not?" With some hesitation but with conviction, Sally remarked with a twinkle in her eyes, "How about talking about me once in a while?" The therapist responded, "Well, how about talking about me once in a while?"

> Sally rebutted, "You just don't understand kids! Don't you know you look like Marlon Brando? Mommy and I are always having fights about him and we say that you look like him." Sally could then turn to a meaningful discussion of her oedipal transference, forbidden sexual thoughts, and masturbatory guilt.

In dealing with his transference neurosis, the adolescent often chooses to displace his feelings and fantasies onto a different object. To ward off the dangers induced in the therapeutic situation, the patient selects an object that is safe--more distant, usually unattainable and unavailable. Only when the patient develops a sufficient degree of self-confidence and adaptive resourcefulness through a discussion of the distant object, can he deal with the transference directly. This is what appears to have happened with Sally.

Certain transference phenomena, such as the belief in the magical power of the therapist, distortions of good and evil, can occasionally be dealt with directly. Paradigmatic psychotherapy utilizes the concept of joining the patient's fantasy to stimulate the verbalization of repressed affects and the uncovering of repressed memories.

> Bob, age 14, a thin, emaciated, easily intimidated youth, extremely withdrawn and asocial, fatherless and friendless, saw the therapist as a God. Despite the transcendental powers of the therapist, in the treatment situation Bob was a bigger God and mocked the therapist at every opportunity. "I know you think you are a big shot, you make lots of dough and read guys' minds but I got your number. I can see through you better than you can see through me." As treatment went on Bob brought in tall stories of his journeys to planets and outer space where he "licked supermen tooth and nail." However, the therapist always responded triumphantly that he had been to these planets many times and in fact had trained Superman. No matter how absurd Bob's fantasy was, the therapist "went him one better." The therapist could climb mightier mountains, swim longer seas, and climb higher trees.

> For over a year-and-a-half this type of interchange prevailed until Bob became quite disgusted and said, "You are a bit of a liar, you know. I bet you never did those things. Most of them are impossible anyway. You really lie a lot. Why do you lie so much?" The therapist asked, "What's wrong with lying?" Bob then gave all the reasons for the therapist's lying. "If you really thought you were a big shot, you wouldn't brag so much. You need a psychologist."
>
> The treatment had begun. Bob could start analyzing the therapist's bizarre fantasies (really his own) and attempt to understand their roots.

The above therapeutic maneuver is described by Anna Freud in The Psychoanalytical Treatment of Children. Children who feel they can do very well without a therapist need an introductory phase where the therapist makes himself interesting. Simultaneously, he becomes aware of the patient's interests and inclinations which lie near the surface.[11]

Particularly when reality is so painful as it was to Bob, described in the above case, the therapist has to respect the patient's distortions until the patient himself "can come down to earth." Robert Lindner's intervention with the patient described in "The Jet Propelled Couch" illuminates this principle.[13]

As is true with many patients in general, and with adolescents in particular, their dependency on the analyst may become so intolerable that the wish to flee from treatment becomes very intense.

> A fifteen-year-old youth, Sam, entered treatment easily and spoke without hesitation of his many conflicts. His father was not available to him so "I kind of like the idea of coming in to talk to somebody like you. I'm depressed a lot and can't concentrate on my schoolwork." Sam found an ego ideal in the person of the therapist, looked forward to his treatment hours, and decided soon after therapy began that he would become a child analyst. After three months of treatment, twice a week, he came in with a pipe for the therapist and said, "This is a present for you.

I'm no longer depressed. As a matter of fact, I feel great. You helped me a lot. I think it is time to quit."

Rather than interpret the patient's transference cure and flight into health, Sam was asked, "When do you want to quit? Now?" Sam, rather surprised at the therapist's response, exclaimed, "Oh, no. At the end of today will be all right." The therapist then wondered why Sam wanted to wait that long. After a long silence, Sam choked up and tearfully remarked, "I can't leave that fast. Let's talk a bit." The more distance the therapist supplied, the closer Sam allowed himself to come. In succeeding hours he could eventually discuss his homosexual anxieties and fear of too much dependence.

Summary and Conclusions

This paper does not purport to be an exhaustive study on adolescence, nor are the case studies intended to be prescriptions for the manifold treatment problems that young patients present. There are many young people exhibiting classical neurotic symptomatology who suffer greatly and can respond very well to more classically-oriented psychotherapy. Often, adolescents find themselves in acute situational maladjustments where several interviews with an understanding adult may be enough to get them over the difficulty. Here, we may refer to decisions about college, the army, or difficulties involving a teacher, employer, girl friend or boy friend.

It has been this writer's experience that severely acting-out youngsters--as were none of the cases described in this paper--usually do not respond to out-patient psychotherapy. Acting-out youngsters often need the sense of security that only residential treatment affords, where their sense of guilt can be more expediently alleviated and where a sanctioned gratification of unconscious dependency needs take place. Many adolescents actually need to be physically separated from their homes where the residential treatment center may ally itself with the healthy parts of the ego in maintaining control and break the vicious cycle between the significant adults of the patient's home life.[3]

For many young people who cannot tolerate a one-to-one relationship where the focus is on themselves, group therapy has proven beneficial. The overdependence on the therapist is obviated as the group therapist encourages the development of relationships with larger groups of people.[27, 13]

In passing, it should be noted that as in the treatment of latency and pre-latency children, parents should be involved in the treatment of the adolescent so that the gains made by the patient can be assimilated and the family balance kept in harmony.[9, 10, 31]

Treatment of the adolescent must maintain at all times a delicate balance between allying itself with the ego or with the instinct. Many analysts who consistently use the classical methods of psychoanalysis have become aware of the need for more subtle intervention when treating the adolescent.[7, 10, 11, 16] Paradigmatic technique reflects an adaptation to the many problems of the adolescent, who frequently responds negatively to classical interpretive intervention. It realizes that "the therapist and the therapeutic situation must provide concomitantly and in nice balance, a dependable relationship and emotional freedom, dependent security and developmental situation, control and ego ideal."[3]

Notes

1. Aichorn, A.: Wayward Youth. New York: Viking Press, 1948.

2. Blos, P.: The Adolescent Personality. New York: Appleton-Century-Croft, 1941.

3. ________: The Treatment of Adolescents. Psychoanalysis and Social Work. ed. Marcel Heiman. New York: International Universities Press, Inc., 1953.

4. Coleman, M. L.: Externalization of the Toxic Introject: A Treatment Technique for Borderline Cases. Psychoanalytic Review, Vol. 43, No. 2, 1956.

5. ________: and B. Nelson: Paradigmatic Psychotherapay in Borderline Treatment. Psychoanalysis, Vol. 5, No. 3, 1957.

6. Eisenstein, V.: Differential Psychotherapy of Borderline States. Specialized Techniques in Psychotherapy. New York: Grove Press, Inc., 1952.

7. Eissler, K. R.: Notes on Problems of Technique in the Psychoanalytic Treatment of Adolescents: With Some Remarks on Perversions. Psychoanalytic Study of the Child, Vol. XIII, New York: International Universities Press.

8. Fairbairn, W. R. D.: An Object-Relations Theory of the Personality. New York: Basic Books, 1954.

9. Feldman, Y.: A Casework Approach Toward Understanding Parents of Emotionally Disturbed Children, Social Work, Vol. III, No. 3, 1958.

10. Freud, A.: The Ego and the Mechanisms of Defense. New York: International Universities Press, 1946.

11. ____________: The Psychoanalytic Treatment of Children: London: Images Publishing Company, 1946.

12. Gitelson, M.: Direct Psychotherapy in Adolescence. American Journal of Orthopsychiatry, Vol. 12, 1942.

13. Greenwald, H.: Great Cases in Psychoanalysis. New York: Ballantine Books, 1959.

14. Hacker, F. J. and E. R. Geleerd: Freedom and Authority in Adolescence. American Journal of Orthopsychiatry, Vol. 14, 1945.

15. Hurlock, E.: The Psychology of Adolescence. New York: McGraw-Hill, 1948.

16. Hoffer, W.: Deceiving the Deceiver, Searchlights on Delinquency. ed. K. R. Eissler. New York: International Universities Press, 1949.

17. Kesten, J.: Learning Through Spite. Psychoanalysis, Vol. 4, No. 1, 1957.

18. Knoepfmacher, L.: Child Guidance Work Based on Psychoanalytic Concepts. The Nervous Child, Vol. 5, No. 2, 1946.

19. Lander, J.: The Pubertal Struggle Against the Instincts. American Journal of Orthopsychiatry, Vol. 12, 1942.

20. Love, S. and H. Mayer: Going Along with Defenses in Resistive Families. Journal of Social Casework, February, 1959.

21. Nagelberg, L.: The Meaning of Help in Psychotherapy. Psychoanalysis and the Psychoanalytic Review, Vol. 46, No. 4, 1959.

22. __________: and H. Spotnitz: Initial Steps in the Analytic Therapy of Schizophrenia in Children. The Quarterly Journal of Child Behavior, Vol. 4, No. 1, January, 1952.

23. __________: and Y. Feldman: The Attempt at Healthy Insulation in the Withdrawn Child. The American Journal of Orthopsychiatry, Vol. 23, No. 2, April, 1953.

24. __________: and H. Spotnitz: Strengthening the Ego Through the Release of Frustration-Aggression. The American Journal of Orthopsychiatry, Vol. 28, No. 4, 1958.

25. Nelson, M. Coleman: Effect of Paradigmatic Techniques on the Psychic Economy of Borderline Patients. Psychiatry (in press).

26. Reichmann, F. Fromm: Notes on the Development of Treatment of Schizophrenics by Psychoanalytic Psychotherapy. Specialized Techniques in Psychotherapy, New York: Grove Press, Inc., 1952.

27. Rosenthal, L.: Some Aspects of a Triple Relation: Activity Group--Group Therapist--Supervisor, New Frontiers in Child Guidance. New York: International Universities Press, 1958.

28. Spotnitz, H., L. Nagelberg and Y. Feldman: Ego Reinforcement in the Schizophrenic Child. The American Journal of Orthopsychiatry, Vol. 26, No. 1, January, 1956.

29. Sternbach, O. and L. Nagelberg: On the Patient-Therapist Relationship in Some 'Untreatable Cases.' Psychoanalysis, Vol. 5, 1957.

30. Strean, H.: The Use of the Patient as Consultant. Psychoanalysis and The Psychoanalytic Review, Vol. 46, No. 2, 1959.

31. ________________: Treating Parents of Emotionally Disturbed Children Through Role Playing. Psychoanalysis and The Psychoanalytic Review, Vol. 47, No. 1, 1960.

32. Wexler, M.: The Structural Problem in Schizophrenia: The Role of the Internal Object. Psychotherapy With Schizophrenics. New York: International Universities Press, 1952.

33. Zwick, P. A.: Gauging Dosage and Distance in Psychotherapy with Adolescents. American Journal of Orthopsychiatry, Vol. 30, No. 3, July, 1960.

8. Reconsiderations in Casework Treatment of the Unmarried Mother

by Herbert S. Strean

Reprinted with permission of the National Association of Social Workers, from Social Work, vol. 13, no. 4, Oct. 1968, p. 91-100.

An historical overview of social work's philosophy about and orientation to the unmarried mother yields several sequential trends. Until the early 1920's virtually the sole concern of the social agency was the unmarried mother's infant and help to the mother herself was rarely considered. As dynamic psychiatry made its inroads and began to influence social work's thinking and activity, the unmarried mother began to be appreciated in her own right and the purposiveness of her behavior was pondered. With the fairly recent advent of ego psychology and the social sciences, the unmarried mother's complete role network--her relationship to various subsystems, e.g., ethnic group, kinship ties, and so on--has become part of the caseworker's psychosocial diagnosis and enriched his treatment plan for her and her child.[1]

Concomitant with the impact of sociology, anthropology, and social psychology on social work has been the intensification of the profession's sense of social responsibility.[2] The cluster of economic, social, psychological, and health variables that are now seen as impinging on the unmarried mother have pointed to a more pressing need for the provision of community resources.[3] While the social planner and policy-maker have presented valid arguments reiterating that effective casework alone cannot be considered the complete answer to the unmarried mother's plight,[4] as Perlman has pointed out, casework is not dead and individualized services will probably always be necessary for some people even if optimum provision of resources could be achieved.[5]

It is incumbent on caseworkers not only to locate where they may legitimately offer their expertise in helping the unmarried mother, but constantly to scrutinize their method and avoid the danger to which Kadushin has pointed, namely, the acceptance of traditional practices in lieu of tested theory.[6] It is the purpose of this paper to evaluate some of the conventional diagnostic hypotheses and classical treatment plans that have evolved in casework with the unmarried mother; certain modifications in casework interventions will be proposed that may more accurately meet certain of the unmarried mother's maturational needs and more expediently enhance certain aspects of her psychosocial functioning.

Review of the Literature

Analysis of the past two decades of social work literature reveals that periodicals in the field have been replete with data on the unmarried mother. Most of the articles have aimed at sensitizing social workers to the subtleties and intricacies of the unmarried mother's personality and/or enriching interventions for her. Virtually every paper or book has begun with the axiom that a multitude of factors contribute to a young woman's becoming pregnant out of wedlock.

Until recently, the search for causes has utilized the metapsychological framework of psychoanalysis and the theme pervading most of the literature in the 1940's and '50's was that the unmarried mother had a conflicted relationship with her own mother and was improperly nurtured at early levels of development. In addition to being the recipient of fragmented mothering, she was seen as having often experienced her father as withdrawn and cold.[7] Common to most of these young women has been an alleged narcissistic character structure, i.e., the girls have been described as extremely preoccupied with their own infantile wishes, which they have had to discharge impulsively. The baby she conceived has frequently been considered to be a narcissistic extension of the unmarried mother and her wish to mother the baby seen as similar to psychologically mothering herself.[8]

The level of ego development of most of these girls has been viewed as "infantile" or "primitive." "They also feel very deprived or depraved."[9] According to most authors, they have not developed mature methods of resolving conflicts and are so self-absorbed that they cannot love others.[10] The young woman has often reported a feeling of being an "ugly duckling" most of her life and conceiving a baby has been in part an attempt to make restitution for her own defects.[11]

The unmarried mother as observed by most psychoanalytically and social work-oriented professionals appears to manifest severe superego lacunae and therefore has been considered delinquent in internalizing societal norms and standards. Not having witnessed in her own home the positive values inherent in a wholesome husband-wife or parent-child relationship, she has been declared incapable of setting standards for her own behavior.[12] Often she has come to the social agency during her fourth or fifth month of pregnancy, seeking specific services; she has tended to withdraw from contact when a plan for the baby has been concluded. Few have taken kindly to the idea of regular casework sessions and if the client has appeared well motivated for continuing treatment, she has been viewed as suspect. The unmarried mother has frequently been described as resistant, defensive, and unresponsive to treatment, usually demanding immediate pragmatic solutions and becoming angry if these are not forthcoming.[13]

The treatment of choice for unmarried mothers has been an ongoing relationship with a female caseworker. Often deserted by the putative father and having experienced emotional abandonment by her own mother, the client allegedly needs "a motherly person who will serve as a refuge during a time of stress."[14] A woman caseworker, it has been concluded, can most appropriately serve as "a healthy object for identification, making it possible [for the client] to accept herself as a woman."[15] Since four out of five unmarried mothers who come to a social agency give the baby up for adoption, it has been alleged that for the mother to give her baby to a woman caseworker is like "making up" with her own mother and thus finalizing a bad experience.[16] (Of the unmarried mothers who do not come to agencies, many do not give their babies up for adoption; of this group, most--especially young Negro women--turn the baby over to their own mothers.[17])

During the last several years the social work field--as reflected in its literature--has slightly altered its focus on the unmarried mother. Instead of concentrating almost exclusively on the client's psychological motives and internal dynamics, the field has been more preoccupied with unmarried motherhood as a social problem, shown more concern for the culture and subculture in which the young woman resides, considered the significant others in her environment, and been quite sensitive to the social values impinging on her.[18] The Negro unmarried mother in particular has received much consideration; she has been reported to be more indifferent and less sensitive to the stigma of illegitimacy because of a greater tolerance of it in her subculture.[19] Although frequently turning over the care of her child to her own mother, the Negro unmarried mother is nonetheless ascribed "an exceptional maternal capacity" and a sexually fertile constitution.[20]

Although the increments to social work's knowledge of the unmarried mother have been substantial and despite valiant attempts on the part of many skilled workers to involve the client in a meaningful casework relationship, as Friedman stated recently, "We are still powerless to alter the script."[21] These clients frequently remain resistant to social work intervention, in many cases seek service but not understanding, usually do not continue treatment after the baby is born, and it has not been uncommon for them to repeat the same experience that brought them to the agency in the first place.[22]

Revised Diagnosis

Re-examination of the literature reported and experimentation in a few selected agencies in the New York and New Jersey area have led to a revised diagnostic picture of the modal unmarried mother. The treatment plan that has evolved in light of this enriched understanding will be presented both theoretically and by case illustrations.

During the year 1966-67 the writer was permitted to read the case records and/or discuss with the caseworker involved procedures utilized in the treatment of fifteen unmarried mothers seen in four different public and private agencies. Seven of these cases were treated either exclusively by a male worker or by a male conjointly with a female caseworker. The remainder were all seen by female workers and served as a control group for this modest pilot study.

Although this study involved a small number of cases and lacked many of the requirements of a rigorous experimental design, our findings prompted us, nevertheless, to question the traditional view of the unmarried mother, namely, that the answer to the riddle of her behavior resides to a large extent in her relationship to her own mother. Careful review and analysis of many cases illustrated in the literature and of those in treatment at the agencies that the researchers selected at random to visit induced us to hypothesize that the aforementioned conventional view regarding the etiology of the unmarried mother's dynamics provides too narrow a focus and results in a premature closure of her dynamic picture as well as of the casework plan for her.

It appears necessary in light of this study to reconsider seriously the entire family gestalt to which the unmarried mother relates. More often than not, the client is not merely caught in the web of an ambivalent, cold mother-daughter relationship, but frequently has been a pawn in a tempestuous marital relationship. More than occasionally, her birth has stimulated much rivalry between her parents, with the mother clinging to her and the father behaving quite seductively. It is frequently the father's seductiveness that has over-stimulated her immature ego and aroused powerful sexual fantasies with which she has found it extremely difficult to cope. As a result, it is not uncommon to find in the histories of unmarried mothers strong prudishness, puritanical attitudes, and other forms of reaction formation defensiveness.[23]

As the power struggle between the girl's parents mounts and she attempts to deal with her divided loyalties, identifying for a time with her mother and then for another period with her father, the potential unmarried mother gradually finds it more and more difficult to fuse and integrate maternal and paternal introjects. She is never quite certain whether she is male or female, and is almost incessantly flirting with each possibility. As adolescence approaches and the need "to prove" herself assumes even more important dimensions, sexual promiscuity becomes one avenue by which to reassure herself of her tenuous femininity.[24]

Quite frequently the girl's parents have separated or become divorced, with the father leaving the home altogether. His absence activates Oedipal and incestuous longings, but because of the girl's recognition of her mother's angry and vitriolic feelings toward her husband, she has to repress and suppress her attachment to her father; she cannot discuss her distress with her mother because of the latter's bias. It is perhaps being left alone with a mother who the young girl feels has deprived her of a father that may account in great measure for what has been referred to as a "pathological and ambivalent mother-daughter relationship." Possibly it is the father's withdrawal that may arouse in the client the self-image of being ugly, "deprived and depraved"--deprived not so much of pregenital and pre-Oedipal love from a mother, but of Oedipal contact with a father; depraved not so much because of a poor maternal object with whom to identify, but because she has been overwhelmed with sexual fantasies and can no longer cathect them in the direction of her sexually exciting but unavailable father. Schmideberg has pointed out: "Many girls became promiscuous during wartime because their fathers were away."[25]

Unwed Mother's Mother

The author does not wish to negate the tremendous influence of the mother in the unmarried mother's development, but rather to appreciate the mother even more--she is not merely an ambivalent object but a figure who enacts many roles and who is relating to many significant others in the client's environment. All of her interactions and transactions are witnessed by her daughter and affect the latter's self-image and attitude toward the world.

In attempting to comprehend more thoroughly the unmarried mother's own mother, many life histories of the latter were studied. It was found that frequently the mother was recapitulating her own life story with her daughter. Often the victim herself of cold, withdrawn, and punitive fathering, she appeared to arrange to live vicariously through her daughter as the latter subtly but sexually interacted with her father. However, out of jealousy and competition with her daughter, who was achieving what she could not, the mother threw roadblocks into the very dyad that she herself had initiated. This does make her an ambivalent object for identification. However, the ambivalent feelings that the unmarried mother feels toward her own mother are nurtured by her fantasies toward her father, which she cannot share with her mother but must rather keep hidden from her. It is these forbidden and secretive sexual impulses toward the father that are often acted out in a clandestine affair; because they are forbidden, they are expressed in a way that will bring punishment.

What should be emphasized is that the girl's resentment toward her mother arose not so much because the latter failed to nurture her properly at early developmental levels, but because the mother has distorted heterosexual attitudes that can only intensify the young girl's conflict. Also of tremendous importance are the client's conflicting feelings toward her father, whom she fantasies as a sexual partner but fears as too engulfing. She is contemptuous of her father because he has not responded maturely as a husband to his wife. If he had been a responsible husband, the girl reasons, then he would have been free enough to relate to his daughter as a growing girl rather than primarily as a sexual object. He has become simultaneously too attractive and too dangerous to his daughter and her developing ego cannot withstand the excruciating dilemma. Therefore, the baby that the unmarried mother conceives is not only the baby that she wishes to be, but often is the fantasied outcome of incest. Is it any wonder that after the product of incest has been born the client does not want to face her mother figure, the caseworker? Her incestuous guilt is too overwhelming, so that at best she turns the baby over to the mother figure to whom she feels it rightfully belongs, and leaves!

In the majority of cases reviewed it was found that when the father withdrew, the mother-daughter relationship, although desired as a refuge by the daughter, became a battleground with both mother and daughter appearing as two immature girls. The mother was seen by her daughter as unable to provide sexual guidance or advice about men or to cater to her maturing sexual interest and questions. Therefore, it has tentatively been concluded that when the young woman appears infantile, demanding, and hyper-dependent in her early casework interviews, this occurs not so much because of a fixation at primitive and infantile levels, but as a regression to earlier modes of satisfaction because present conflicts are too overwhelming and the current environment is not sufficiently supportive.

Most of the mothers studied viewed their teen-age daughters as a potpourri of unintegrated conflicts and impulses with whom a relationship was too burdensome. In several cases the mother herself often turned to sexual affairs as a refuge, frequently looking for "fatherly-type men." As one mother, speaking on her daughter's behalf as well as her own, said: "Neither of us had a good father so we thought we were 'punks' as girls. Getting a guy to 'knock us up' somehow tells us that at least for a while we're O.K." However, because the self-hating impulse has remained active throughout, these women frequently chose men who left them or, if they remained, became insensitive and infantile father figures.

The absence of the father altogether or the presence of a father who deprives his daughter of the satisfaction of being a girl (and not just a sexual object) seems to appear where unmarried motherhood occurs must frequently, namely, among lower socioeconomic Negro families. The girl during the course of her development has usually had some relationships with older men that have frequently been tantalizing, but the consistent unavailability of a mature father figure is ubiquitous. Certainly the host of attendant economic and other social variables inherent in the Negro constellation should not or cannot be minimized; it is, nonetheless, a virtual truism that unmarried motherhood is prevalent in circumstances in which the father is unavailable.[26]

While the importance of the father in a girl's psychosocial development has in general been relatively undefined and the effects of paternal deprivation largely unspecified, we are beginning to become sensitized to the uniquely paternal contributions necessary for a girl's development as she shifts from primary to secondary dependency. As Forrest has pointed out, for a female to be fulfilled as a person and a woman, the father's presence from infancy through childhood, girlhood, and adolescence aids and abets psychological growth.[27]

How Help Is Offered

Because it has been tentatively hypothesized that part of the etiology of the unmarried mother's difficulty is the absence of mature fathering, that the quest for "pre-Oedipal mothering" on her part stems more from a regression to old modes of functioning than from a fixation, and that the client's mother is so flooded with anxiety of her own that renders her incapable of meeting her daughter's maturational needs--especially the need to see her mother function in mature heterosexual relationships--it is proposed that casework intervention must seek to meet these unmet needs.

Is it not possible that the way the unmarried mother experiences casework help as it is presently structured for her may recapitulate the ugly experiences that brought her to the agency in the first place? More than nine times out of ten she is confronted by a female worker who initially wishes to "understand" her rather than immediately give her tangibles, such as advice and information about the baby's delivery and the external factors attending it. What the client usually wants from the caseworker initially, namely, informative advice, is what her mother could not give her. When her initial requests are subjected to study rather than immediately met, she does become "demanding and hostile." If the hostility is not seen as a defensive response to the hurt and anguish the client is feeling because no one cares about her, the kind of power struggle that transpired with her own mother might ensue with the caseworker.

Another feature of the way help is offered to the unmarried mother that repeats past traumas is the absence of a man in the treatment plan. Occasionally the putative father is interviewed if available and sometimes the client's own father is approached, but most social agencies working with unmarried mothers, especially group residences, have a completely female atmosphere. While the less traditional agencies and more modern caseworkers have inaugurated casework plans that include the few men in the girl's life (and with good results), it is the author's finding that this is more the exception than the rule.[28] When a male worker, trained or untrained, becomes part of the treatment plan and if in addition significant men in the girl's environment are sought out, the casework experience for the unmarried mother comes closer to meeting her psychosocial deprivations. Because, according to the writer's data, the most fundamental lacuna in the unmarried mother's ego development has been the lack of men and women working together in her behalf, it is this latter experience, if planfully utilized as part of work with her, that can improve the casework results appreciably.

Suggested Treatment Model

In several cases by plan and in some cases by accident the following structured approach has been found to be most beneficial in casework treatment of the unmarried mother:

1. Because the unmarried mother comes to an agency in a state of crisis and panic that has been precipitated by her illegitimate pregnancy and frequently exacerbated by her mother's anxiety, her father's withdrawal, and the putative father's emotional and often physical isolation, she will inevitably conduct herself in a regressed, infantile and demanding manner. The female caseworker rather than making interpretations about the client's behavior or asking questions in an attempt to clarify her motives, should try to answer her questions immediately. Initially, information should not be provided about agency practice and policy unless the client asks for this; rather, she should be given information that _she wants for herself._ As the client is "given to" in terms of what she wants, the worker is gradually experienced as the nurturing mother who has her psychological daughter's best interests in mind and is genuinely relating to them.

2. With the caseworker's demonstration of concern about matters pertaining to the client's physical case--who the doctor will be, diet, medical prescriptions, appropriate exercises, details of the delivery, and so on--the client usually begins to become more interested in the worker as a person. As a result, she begins to share with the worker the experiences that brought her to the agency, her confusion regarding sexual matters, and her debilitating experiences with her parents. She often comes up with a statement or

question that disguises, yet implies, a cry for help as if casework treatment were to begin only now (although contacts have transpired for several weeks). The wish for help is usually couched in statements about her poor self-image and her desire to be rid of it. As the caseworker relates to the client's formulation of her own problems and concerns, the idea of treatment or counseling can be discussed meaningfully and nondefensively by both worker and client.

3. At this stage a male worker should be introduced to the client for counseling. The rationale for this proposal should be explained to the client as follows: "I agree that your relationships with men have caused you a lot of difficulty. I think, therefore, that it would be helpful for you if you had a male caseworker. As you learn to get along with him, I'm quite sure that you'll be able to get along with many other men in the future."

The client initially interprets this proposal to mean that the female caseworker will be "dropping out of the picture." The caseworker should explain: "On the contrary, I'll be around whenever you need me. You are still concerned about doctors, nurses, hospital visits, and the like, and I'm here to help you with these concerns." Invariably, after two or three interviews the client's response is euphoric and ecstatic: "You mean I'll have you both. That's great!"

4. The opportunity to work with a male worker and not lose the female worker offers the client the opportune situation of which she has been deprived. Given a non-seductive male and a mother figure who is genuinely concerned increases the self-image positively, mobilizes previously intact ego functions, and frequently enables the client to reflect genuinely on herself and her interaction with her environment, present and past.

5. The triadic relationship continues after the birth of the infant and as long as the client needs it. In addition, if the girl's father, mother, or the baby's putative father can be part of the treatment plan, the client feels far from alone but instead enjoys "all the attention I am getting."

6. From time to time, and dictated by the client's

needs and requests, both male and female workers see her together. The rationale for this maneuver is explained as follows: "We want you to have the opportunity really to experience a man and a woman working together in your behalf."

Experimentation has been done not only with trained workers but with untrained workers as well. Given appropriate supervision, it has been found that persons with only undergraduate education can adapt to the cited approach, provided it is well structured in advance so that salient client responses can be anticipated and appropriate interventions timed accordingly. The six steps enumerated appear to offer the client an emotionally corrective experience with an unambivalent mother figure and a nonseductive father figure. The treatment is designed to meet the developmental needs of the unmarried mother--to feed her when she needs emotional nourishment, to educate her when she needs information and knowledge, and to offer her fatherly admiration and maternal tenderness when these are required.

Case Illustrations

Miss A, a young Negro woman of 31, had five illegitimate pregnancies. Living in a housing project and on welfare, she was frequently drunk, often depressed, and managed her home and children with extremely limited care and discipline. The management of the project sent a female case aide--an untrained worker--to "see what could be done" before processing an eviction.

The worker found Miss A's house extremely untidy, her children poorly cared for, and Miss A in the third month of her sixth pregnancy. The case aide told Miss A that the management of the project had suggested that she be seen, but before the worker could finish her opening remarks, the client bellowed: "Oh, they want to throw me out because they don't like the way I keep the house!" The worker looked around and said calmly: "I'm sure things are very difficult for you. You must have it very rough." The client spent the next half hour talking about how her children were a burden to her, that meeting their physical needs was impossible, how difficult it was to make ends meet financially, and that the only pleasure she got once in a while was "a little sex and a little drink." The worker remarked that she could understand how sex and drinking could be her only pleasures but wondered if there was anything that she, the worker, could do to bring her some pleasure. Miss A pointed to the children's clothes and her poor furniture, and mentioned that she had limited time for herself. The worker immediately responded: "I'll get in touch with a few places and people and see what can be done."

The worker did get in touch with the department of welfare and other agencies in the community in order to supply Miss A with some of the tangibles she requested. Therefore, with some physical needs met--clothes for the children and mother, mattresses and beds, and a volunteer for some babysitting--the client began, in her second interview, to talk about her current pregnancy and previous ones as well. She said that she knew "damn well that I don't appeal to men" and that all of her sexual affairs turned out to be one-night stands. When the worker took note of the client's feelings of depreciation vis-à-vis men, and said: "You think that the only reason men would have anything to do with you is to go to bed, don't you?" Miss A tearfully reported how she remembered as a little girl wishing that a boy friend of her mother's who intermittently visited the house "could be my father." She then spent some time talking about her wish for a father who "would have really cared about me" but how her mother "just didn't meet up with a good man to live with."

As Miss A continued to talk about her feelings of deprivation in her heterosexual relationship, the worker gradually introduced the subject of a male worker, who was part of the same social service department of the housing project. Miss A did not ask for any explanation of the entrance of the male worker into the situation but seemed to sense the rationale behind the introduction and merely said; "Great!"

In contrast to the manner in which Miss A usually cared for the house, the male worker at his first interview found it to be extremely tidy and the children and Miss A well groomed. This held true at subsequent visits. While Miss A continued to see the female worker about plans for the baby and dealt with the situation quite responsibly, with the male worker she talked about the possibility of working, which he encouraged. Through his efforts, Miss A took a job in the postoffice, did excellent work there (enough to receive part of a maternity leave with pay), and talked with both of her workers about the new "but different" men in her life who "seem to respect me."

While a case situation like Miss A's will remain open for some time and Miss A will see both workers intermittently, at one interview she explained the modifications in her life by saying: "I got a good mommy and daddy--that's all you need to feel good!"

* * *

Miss L., a 19-year-old Jewish girl, came to a family agency during her fourth month of pregnancy. Referred by a physician, she blurted out in her first intake interview: "I want to give up my baby for adoption." The female caseworker immediately responded: "Then I think you've come to the right place. That's our business here; maybe we can help you!" The client, a little surprised, said: "Good, I thought you'd want to ask me a bunch of personal questions!" The worker responded; "Oh, I thought *you'd* want to ask *me* a bunch of questions!" The client stated that she did, and asked many pertinent questions about hospital delivery, seeing the baby, nurses, residence, and so on, all of which the worker answered directly, truthfully, and factually. Miss L gladly initiated a second appointment with the same worker, and on leaving said: "Enjoyed it!"

Miss L arrived on time for her second appointment and within a few minutes volunteered without prompting the details of her pregnancy and of previous relationships with young men. She was able to say: "I know I've used sex to make me feel adequate. I guess I've wondered most of my life how much of a female I am!" When the intake worker asked her how she accounted for her "feeling of inadequacy," Miss L described her relationships with her parents. According to her, her mother was extremely con-concerned with her own appearance and "always squabbled with my father." Her father was described as a "sensitive and passionate man," who "used to tickle me a lot." Further references to Miss L's father led the worker to help her focus on the highly stimulating experiences with him and the longings she felt for him when her parents separated when she was 16. On her own, Miss L dated her sexual acting out with her father's leaving home.

Miss L participated actively in the intake interviews and eventually requested treatment. She was assigned a male worker to whom she eagerly remarked in the first interview: "I need to see a man counselor so that I can get along with men better." Rather quickly she attempted to initiate a mutually seductive relationship with the worker. When he pointed this out to her, she experienced it as a rejection, saying quite pitifully: "No men like me," and recalled relationships with young men in which she felt abandonment and rejection. The worker responded: "Just because it wouldn't be good for treatment for me to have sex with you doesn't mean I want to leave you!" The treatment became quite challenging for Miss L at this point. She found it difficult to believe that a man would like her and yet not go to bed with her. Here the worker was able to say: "If we weren't more interested in seeing you get help it might be fun," thus demonstrating to her that a father figure could have sexual feelings but could control them.

Miss L continued her treatment after the baby was born. The worker was able to involve both of her parents in the delivery and adoption proceedings. Interestingly, Miss L's father asked for treatment himself and was referred for private psychotherapy. The female worker Miss L saw at intake was utilized at strategic times during the process--once when Miss L wanted information about gynecological matters and another time when Miss L was thinking about attending a college that was the worker's alma mater.

Miss L visited both workers after she left the community and went away to college. Eventually she became interested in a career in social work.

Summary and Conclusion

Examination of the social work literature on the unmarried mother and investigation of cases in selected agencies led to the conclusion that the dynamic formulations that have placed the prime etiological factor in the mother-daughter relationship required modification and further elaboration. While the importance of pre-Oedipal nurturing in the mother-daughter relationship should not be discounted in the study, diagnosis, or treatment of the unmarried mother, it was proposed that the client must be viewed within her total family constellation. Important, therefore, is the unmarried mother's perception of her parents' interaction as well as her unique relationship to her father.

De-emphasized in the literature has been the importance of the father's contribution to the unmarried mother's sexual difficulties. His seductiveness and eventual withdrawal were seen as prime factors in the development of the girl's difficulties. The question was raised as to whether the prevalence of unmarried motherhood in certain subcultures may be due, in part, to a high incidence of absence of the father.

A structured treatment plan involving male and female workers who would offer the unmarried mother a corrective emotional experience was presented along with case illustrations.

Notes

1. See Jane K. Goldsmith, "The Unmarried Mother's Search for Standards," Social Casework, Vol. 48, No. 2 (February 1957), p. 69-73; and Vera Shlakman, "Unmarried Parenthood: An Approach to Social Policy," Social Casework, Vol. 47, No. 8 (October 1966), p. 491-502.
2. Herbert H. Aptekar, "Education for Social Responsibility," Journal of Education for Social Work, Vol. 2, No. 2 (Fall 1966), p. 5-11
3. Martin Wright, "Comprehensive Services for Adolescent Unwed Mothers," Children, Vol. 13 No. 5 (September-October 1966), p. 171-176.
4. See Aptekar, op. cit.
5. Helen Harris Perlman, "Casework Is Dead," Social Casework, Vol. 48, No. 1 (January 1967), p. 22-25.
6. Alfred Kadushin, "The Knowledge Base of Social Work," in Alfred J. Kahn, ed., Issues in American Social Work (New York: Columbia University Press, 1959), p. 39-79.

7. See A. Ferdinand Bonan, "Psychoanalytic Implications in Treating Unmarried Mothers with Narcissistic Character Structures," Social Casework, Vol. 44, No. 6 (June 1963), p. 323-330; and Joseph E. Lifschutz, Theodosia B. Stewart, and Ada M. Harrison, "Psychiatric Consultation in the Public Assistance Agency," Social Casework, Vol. 39, No. 1 (January 1958), p. 3-8.

8. Bonan, op. cit.; Jane G. Judge, "Casework with the Unmarried Mother in a Family Agency," Social Casework, Vol. 32 No. 1 (January 1951), p. 7-14.

9. Bonan, op. cit.

10. Lifschutz, Stewart, and Harrison, op. cit.

11. Judge, op. cit.

12. Goldsmith, op. cit.

13. Rose Bernstein, "The Maternal Role in the Treatment of Unmarried Mothers," Social Work, Vol. 8, No. 1 (January (1963), p. 58-65; and Bernstein, "Are We Still Stereotyping the Unmarried Mother?" Social Work, Vol. 5 No. 3 (July 1960), p. 22-28.

14. Peter Blos, On Adolescence (New York: Free Press, 1961), p. 27-28.

15. Lifschutz, Stewart, and Harrison, op. cit., p. 50.

16. Helen L. Friedman, "The Mother-Daughter Relationship: Its Potential in Treatment of Young Unwed Mothers," Social Casework, Vol. 47, No. 8 (October 1966), p. 502-507.

17. Wright, op. cit.

18. Ibid.; Shlakman, op. cit.; and Sidney Furie, "Birth Control and the Lower-Class Unmarried Mother," Social Work, Vol. 11, No. 1 (January 1966), p. 42-49.

19. Bernstein, "The Maternal Role in the Treatment of Unmarried Mothers," and "Are We Still Stereotyping the Unmarried Mother?"

20. Bernstein, "The Maternal Role in the Treatment of Unmarried Mothers."

21. Ibid.

22. Frances H. Scherz, "'Taking Sides' in the Unmarried Mother's Conflict," *Social Casework,* Vol. 28, No. 2 (February 1947), p. 57-60.

23. Bonan, *op. cit.*

24. Blos, *op. cit.*

25. Melitta Schmideberg, "Psychiatric-Social Factors in Young Unmarried Mothers," *Social Casework,* Vol. 32, No. 1 (January 1951), p. 3-7.

26. Wright, *op. cit.*

27. Tess Forrest, "Paternal Roots of Female Character Development," *Contemporary Psychoanalysis,* Vol. 3 No. 1 (Fall 1966), p. 21-31.

28. Francis L. Feldman and Frances H. Scherz, *Family Social Welfare: Helping Troubled Families* (New York: Atherton Press, 1967), p. 386.

9. Modifications in Therapeutic Technique in the Group Treatment of Delinquent Boys

by Morris Black and Leslie Rosenthal

It has been stated by Slavson[9] that

> . . . the sine qua non for success in psychotherapy is the proper matching of the type of patient and the type of treatment to be employed. It is from this discriminative choice of suitable procedures made on the basis of clinical considerations, character structure, the nature and source of the patient's disturbances and maladjustments, his life-setting and his life-aims, that therapeutic effectiveness flows. In both group psychotherapy and in individual treatment individuation of approach and process is essential.

This paper deals with changes in therapeutic technique which were instituted to cope with certain difficulties in the group therapy of delinquent, lower-class, Negro male adolescents. We shall present modifications of conventional therapeutic technique which were, of necessity, adapted to a group of youngsters for whom distrust and suspicion were vitally needed defensive attitudes and whose symptoms were ego-syntonic[1, 3-5, 7] and reinforced by their life experiences. Since the literature reported limited therapeutic success, on an out-patient basis, with patients such as these, experimental modifications of technique were deemed necessary.

The group was established in 1961 through the Jewish Board of Guardians' liaison with the Inter-Departmental Neighborhood Service Center (a city agency working with families in one of the highest delinquency areas of New York City) for service to a number of adolescent Negro youngsters. In evaluating the referral material it was our impression that none of the youngsters appeared to show a good prognosis for conventional treatment methods. They all exhibited a high degree of emotional disturbance with severe anti-social symptomatology, e.g., stealing, delinquent gang involvement, truancy, aggressive behavior with teachers and peers, and defiant and negative behavior at home. Other symptoms included learning problems, sibling rivalry, and fearfulness. Diagnostically, the youngsters covered a wide range--from passive-aggressive character disorder, to borderline schizophrenic, or psychotic. Youngsters showing neuroses or neurotic character disorders were not referred. In every instance, symptoms were ego-syntonic with no observable manifest anxiety. Motivation for treatment was either minimal or non-existent.

Each of the five youngsters in the group came from neighborhoods characterized by a complex of unfavorable conditions for living associated with slums: high crime rate, adult criminality, delinquency, drug addiction, prostitution, and racketeering. In the typical familial constellation we found a two-fold deprivation: 1) a mother whose nurturing care of the baby was quickly interrupted by environmental pressures and who reacted to the male infant with hostility and rejection and 2) the complete absence of a father or the presence of a series of inadequate father surrogates.

Abandonments, both real and symbolic, dominated the life experiences of these boys. As a consequence of disrupted, distorted, primary object relationships, the development of their egos, of adequate self-images, of a solid sense of sexual identity, and of a capacity for meaningful object relations, were impaired. As expected, the real and psychological unavailability of the mother and the absence of a consistent, stable father resulted in underdeveloped and primitive super-egos.

The most compelling characteristic of these boys was pervasive distrust. In view of this, we felt that subjecting them to classical intake procedures would result in our losing them in the intake process, particularly as the group therapist was white. Therefore, the group therapist himself conducted a brief initial screening interview with each boy prior to the beginning of the group. In these interviews, the therapist talked about the group as being an experimental one and stated that he did not know whether he or the group could help them. The choice of joining was left to the boy, although it was made clear that the family case worker from the Inter-Departmental Neighborhood Service Center would be in touch with the therapist while they were in the group. Throughout the life of the group, the therapist maintained constant contact with the INSC worker, an "untrained" worker who attempted to deal with the multiple economic, medical and legal needs of the youngsters and their families.

In the beginning, the boys needed some external pressure to insure that they would come to group sessions. Often, the family worker would fulfill this function by visiting the youngsters' homes to supply them with carfare to get to the group or to actually bring them. We felt that the group therapist should not put himself in the position whereby the youngsters would feel that he was making them come to the group. We felt that the boys would interpret the group therapist's desire to help or to change them as his wanting to "con" or manipulate them for his own needs. We also believed that on another level the boys would react to him as a threat to their precariously achieved ego-equilibrium.

In the planning stages of the group we debated the suitability of an interview (verbal method) as against a motorically centered form of activity group therapy. The decision was made to use verbal group methods based upon our belief that it would not be fair to pre-judge their ability to convey feelings in language rather than in action, and that an action-oriented group might constitute an infantilization of these 14 to 16 year-old boys. Even though we were not sure that this would be successful, we decided to try it. If the anxiety level rose too high, we were prepared to introduce arts and crafts material as diluting agents. While we were uncertain as to which specific therapeutic technique should be used, we had great doubt that conventional group analytic technique could be applied in an unmodified form because these youngsters had such great difficulty in verbalizing rather than in expressing themselves in action. It was apparent that these boys could not accept the basic premise of therapy, because of their distrust, that the therapist has a right to explore and to question the patient. The group was thus conceived in an atmosphere of distrust on the part of the group members and therapeutic uncertainty on the part of the authors.

Resistance

In starting, the therapist described the purpose and activity of the group as "getting things off your chests," telling the story of their lives, and putting their feelings into words. We restricted ourselves to the barest minimum of rules: no hitting other group members or running through the halls. We viewed their delinquent, antisocial activity as being, on one level symptomatic of psychological disturbance but, more importantly, as being a reflection of their learned, and even adoptive behavior. Therefore we related to such behavior largely in terms of seeking further understanding of it.

As was to be expected, the group members resisted doing what the therapist outlined to them as the work of the group. Rather than talking, they engaged in motor activity, especially in the early life of the group. They sought to immobilize the therapist by threatening him with physical attack and they acted out in the building after sessions by running up and down the halls, provoking secretaries and maintenance personnel, running the elevator up and down and attacking the weaker group members. There was also a marked discontinuity of discussion in that the group almost compulsively darted from one subject to another without being able to focus for any sustained period on any one theme. This pattern may well have reflected the instability in their own lives and the fact that they were never the recipients of more than transitory and flitting emotional interest and attention themselves. This pattern imposed quite a demand on the therapist for emotional flexibility and agility.

Contrary to the course of events in many other groups, the members did not curb each other's resistive behavior in the group. At times members made accurate and telling observations about dangerous or self-destructive activities being engaged in by fellow members <u>outside</u> the group: these observations however were never accompanied by demands for change.

Two identifiable group resistances employed by the members were:

1) Resistance derived from the repetition compulsion. Thus the group members sought to induce the therapist to reject, abandon and

alienate himself from them as they had been rejected, abandoned and alienated.

2) The craving for excitement. This was evidenced in their excited talk of aggression, gang wars, etc.

Group Reaction to Food

We decided, as a means of conveying empathy with the intense oral deprivations in the lives of the group members, that refreshments would be offered at group sessions. The food quickly became the nucleus of the group's emotionality. The members showed preoccupation and intense absorption with the kinds of refreshment, the amount, the method of serving and division. Indicative of the strategic role that the refreshments occupied in the life of the group was the comment by one boy, after another youngster had talked about a gang threatening to kill him, was, "Good, now we can have more cake." The other youth exclaimed, "If I'm going to die, it won't be until after I eat at the Christmas party next week." During the first year of the group's existence, there was marked excitement while and after eating, with the youngsters punching holes in the soda cans, squeezing them or beating them on the table. We gradually saw a decrease in such activity as the boys became more and more able to sit and talk. This general pattern continued through the second year. The duration of excitement diminished, there was less need for motor discharge, and a greater tolerance for talking. It was during this later period that Charlie, a highly resistant, hostile, youngster, commented several times after eating, "Okay, we got the grit, now we can talk."

Orality and Ambivalence

Orality was one of the most important dynamic themes and feeling constellations that stood out in the life of the group. There was a tremendous craving to be fed, both concretely and symbolically. Emerging concomittantly with the orality was intense ambivalence toward the feeding person, in this case, the group therapist. Being fed generated anticipation of <u>not</u> being adequately fed which in turn, aroused intense aggressive impulses. In the group, the possibility of frustration evoked threats of murder and dismemberment of the therapist. Another significant feeling complex revolved around the danger of accepting the food. One boy, half seriously, with a can opener against the therapist's neck, warned him that: "If you don't bring two cakes next time instead of one, I'll cut your throat." Steve then added, "Yes, we'll throw you out the window." Another, after grabbing the piece of cake left for the therapist, said, "You're probably wishing we'd all get killed because you really wanted that piece of cake." In addition, the very feeding evoked a whole host of barely suppressed murderous, cannibalistic, and oral-sadistic thoughts and feelings.[6] Steve, talked about how he suddenly realized why the therapist had, several months previously, taken a smaller piece of cake than the others. He felt that the therapist had been systematically poisoning the cake and was therefore taking a smaller piece.

Another example of oral-aggressive impulses was presented when one youngster reported a dream about a rat coming and eating all the children in his block. He also, while doodling, made a drawing of the therapist rising from the grave with a rat in his mouth. In subsequent drawings he showed the therapist as a person with shark's teeth who literally ate people.

We also saw the extensive use of projection as a defense to enable them to cope with their oral ambivalence. We believe that the intensity of the deprivation that was experienced by these youngsters resulted, during their crucial beginning years, in feelings of murderous rage and anger towards the depriving person or object. The young child is extremely frightened by these feelings which, if he were to express them, could potentially result in his own destruction, in retaliation, or in cessation of what little he is receiving. During these formative years there are oral-cannibalistic and oral-sadistic thoughts and fantasies in which the child experiences a feeling of "I kill and I eat." The potential threat of retribution by the object is so terrifying that the child needs to separate himself from these feelings by saying, "These are not my impulses, it's the others who are thinking this; I'm not this kind of person."

In these children we see the development of projection as a major mode of defense against the anxiety created by powerful, burgeoning, aggressive impulses. The harsh realities of their lives offer a realistic validity to the use of this defense.

Walter Miller, in his article "Focal Concerns of Lower-Class Culture,"[7] describes factors which are emphasized among the lower-classes. He stresses the importance of "masculinity," i.e., physical prowess, skill, fearlessness, bravery, daring, the ability to outsmart, and to "con." Seen as a positive attitude is "autonomy which is construed as freedom from external constraint and superordinate authority."[5]

In relating this to the children under discussion we feel that in an environment where there is a good deal of violence and acting out of impulse, the child often does not receive help in learning to control his frightening and destructive, aggressive, impulses. Thus certain adaptive modes of defense become more urgent such as the development of the use of projection described above. In structural terms these children develop and perpetuate a primitive super-ego, in which a hostile and destructive self-image is interjected. At the same time, he projects onto others his own self-image and hostile, destructive, impulses. This is expressed in such attitudes as: "Everyone in the world is out to 'con' everybody else in one way or another; I don't trust adults, nobody trusts anyone."

The child thus develops an acute fear and distrust of others because of the perceived potential danger of attack. He attempts to master his anxiety and to cope with his environment, his aggression, rage, and feelings of emptiness by repetitively keeping up a running battle with "authority," i.e., adults, school and police. The mechanism of projection becomes for such children, not only necessary psychologically, but also an appropriate response to real external threats. In our work with these children we tried to deal with the psychological component within this context.

The struggle to cope with the inner feelings of tension, boredom, restlessness, and vague depression is a never-ending one. The youngster has to constantly be alert to guard against the full impact of his own murderous rage and impulses. He therefore continually has a need to perceive and relate to his problems as external and environmental. A joke told by one of the youngsters in the group might best illustrate their view of the world: Steve told about a man dying and going to heaven. St. Peter welcomes him and then asks, "But why do you have a knife in the coffin?" The man responds, "Man, wherever you are you always need some protection." So entrenched is their distrust that they plan to take it with them to the hereafter! This is a familiar mechanism which serves the purpose of maintaining and reinforcing their perception of the world as hostile, angry, ungiving, and potentially retaliatory. Such children unconsciously attempt to provoke others to react with anger, hostility, and resentment when reality doesn't conform with their projected image of it. When the therapist talked about this, Brian said, "You probably feel you want to throw me out of the group because of all the trouble I've caused here. I've 'intuit-ed' that from the beginning."

Unfortunately, it is not too difficult, in our society, for these youngsters to find grounds for perpetuating this negative self-image and distorted view of the world.

To recapitulate, we found ourselves dealing with a group of boys who showed disturbance in their capacity for object relationships. We saw intense fears of closeness and an inability to trust as related to early maternal deprivation. There was constant preoccupation on the part of these boys in terms of giving and taking, feeding and being fed. Although they wanted very much to be fed, they were extremely ambivalent towards the feeding person. Their fears of intimacy, distrust of others, their use of externalization and projection, their desire for immediate gratification, and need for motor discharge find acceptance in the life experiences of these youngsters. We might speculate that many of the problems and symptoms these boys exhibited were ego-syntonic on a psychological level and "culture-syntonic" on an environmental level, since many of their ideas and impulses were functional and adaptive to survival needs.

Changes in Therapeutic Technique

Analytic group psychotherapy[8] fosters transference, catharsis, insight, and ego-strengthening, reality-testing, and sublimation. As the group developed, and although we had not conceived of this as a typical analytic psychotherapy group, it became apparent that many of the basic elements of analytic group psychotherapy were present. We saw expressions of transference feelings toward the therapist and toward other group members. It became increasingly clear that "feeding" of the boys evoked responses and patterns of behavior which could be directly related to experiences in their own families. Each of the boys spent his energy fighting for the therapist's "food" and attention as he had had to fight at home for what little the mother or father had to give. The ambivalence about the feeding person and about being fed, as well as the ambivalent feelings toward the other group members stood out in sharp relief. The therapy group became quite openly a symbolic approximation of their own families with the group members being seen as siblings and the group therapist as the feeding, ambivalently-regarded mother. After a period of time, the productions of the group members indicated a modification of the maternal transference as the therapist began to emerge as a paternal figure. In response to this development, we attempted to provide a structure in which the boys could test their own projected images of a father while the therapist attempted to project a different kind of father-image. We felt that the therapist ought to provide a primary model for introjection and identification so as to help the boys modify their projections of the "bad" father. The therapeutic task then became one of enabling the youngsters to feel and to express their feelings toward the good and bad father and to aid them in integrating this split image.

Modifications of therapeutic technique evolved from our continued study of the group's resistances and from our attempt to set up a special situation in which the therapeutic tasks of catharsis, insight and ego-building, reality-testing, and sublimation could take place. Spotnitz, in a paper[9] on the borderline schizophrenic in group psychotherapy succinctly states what we conceived of as our own therapeutic task. He says, "The primary emphasis is placed on meeting these two basic needs: first, the need for psychological nourishment in the form of emotional communication or attitude; secondly, adequate psychological release for the high accumulations of destructive or libidinal energy in the mental apparatus of the borderline schizophrenic. <u>Adequate</u> nourishment and <u>adequate</u> release are specified because <u>too</u> much or too <u>little of either</u> one is not therapeutic for this type of patient." In attempting to find a balance between such "adequate" release and nourishment we instituted the following special modifications in therapeutic technique.

Therapeutic Use of Food

Children develop warmth, a capacity for reciprocal relatedness and trust, within the confines of a family where there is some appropriate balance of gratification and frustation. We found in the serving of food that the problems the boys exhibited around impulse control and low frustration tolerance came out to a marked degree in the area of feeding within the group setting. In addition, the serving of food evoked strong sibling rivalry and transference phenomena. We therefore used the feeding as one of our primary therapeutic tools. The youngsters were asked to choose the food for the following week as well as for special occasions. The therapist could not always meet their requests, particularly around parties, where there were requests for enormous and unrealistic quantities of food. On several occasions when the therapist permitted himself to over-feed the group, they complained about being sick and expressed regurgitative impulses. The refreshment situation brought into sharp focus the various roles adopted by the members. For instance, one fearful, withdrawn youngster continually surrendered his turn to cut the cake--a job much desired by the other members. This reflected the boy's denial of his dependency needs as well as his self-derogation. The therapist addressed himself to this by stating, "Walter doesn't seem to feel he's entitled to cut the cake." Subsequently, Walter was able to express his needs and have them met. As the boys sat around the table eating, the familial situation was re-enacted. Life-long adaptational patterns were viewed with a frankness that helped the boys become sensitized to their feelings around nurturance, deprivation, intimacy, and competitiveness. In a sense, the group was like a stage upon which each enacted the dramas of his life history.

Planful Use of the Therapist's Own Feelings

There were two ways in which the therapist used his own feelings. On the one hand, he used them as a demonstration, to the group, that it is permissible to have and express feelings without becoming overwhelmed by them and without relinquishing his strength. On the other hand, they were used to enhance the therapist's own understanding of what the group members were feeling. In view of the fact that to these youngsters, denial of certain universal feelings was pervasive, it was neither psychologically nor culturally comfortable for them to admit such feelings as sadness, fear and grief. In a sense, they had to be trained and helped to feel that they were entitled to these feelings. This re-educative process was so hard for them that it required the group therapist's "demonstrating" these feelings to them, with himself as an example. We learned that the youngsters only responded with their own feelings when the therapist was free enough to give a concrete, emotional demonstration of his own ability and willingness to do so. On one occasion the therapist initiated a session by relating how sad he was that day. This allowed them to experience the sadness, grief and rage they had felt over their own lost love-objects. In another session a youngster talked about his involvement in a gang fight and the threats he had received about being "burned" (shot). He denied any fear about this. The therapist handled this first by giving an "educational talk" about the mechanism of denial in psychology, but this was not very successful and it was only after the therapist admitted fear, in a realistically fear-inducing situation, that they were able to acknowledge their own fear about gang fighting in their neighborhoods, threats of being "burnt," etc. One member could only admit to having cried after discovering that the therapist had himself cried on occasions as an adult. This youngster then related how he had cried two years before, when he had been "busted" (arrested) for stealing clothes in a department store. This was the first time he had talked about any delinquent behavior, and he talked with real feeling about his crying. In effect the therapist was illustrating that it is permissible for a man to have these feelings and still be a man.

Induced Feelings

We also attempted to understand the feelings of frustration, anxiety, impotence, excitement, sadness, and anger experienced by the therapist in working with this group. It was our belief that the group members induced in him certain feelings they themselves had experienced and could not express directly. When the group was unresponsive to the therapist, the deprivation he then felt afforded him an emotional glimpse of the life-long deprivation to which they had been subjected. There were many sessions where the youngsters did not show up or deliberately excluded the therapist from the ongoing group discussion.

On one occasion Charlie commented "who asked you to say anything?" There were many provocative, hostile, and derogatory remarks about the therapist's appearance and behavior as well as repeated threats to throw him out the window or to kill him. We felt that these represented, in part, attempts to symbolically eliminate the therapist by abandoning him first (that is, before he could abandon them) and attempting to provoke him to "abandon" them. This concept was particularly helpful to us during those times when the therapist felt like terminating the group because of his frustration over the lack of response and his resentment at the intense hostility directed against him by the group.

Conventionally, the group therapist hopes for the development of group cohesion, feelings of group belongingness, intra-group rapport, sharing, and mutual support. However, these youngsters seemed to regard this as emotional dynamite. In a sense, such emotional prosperity was too rich for their blood. The therapist had to frustrate his own needs for a warm, close, happy family (group), which ran counter to his whole prior training. We had to learn to respect their defenses of isolation, their needs to retain attitudes or suspicion and distrust, for as long as they were psychologically necessary. Thus, we had to adjust and bear the frustration of the therapist's emotional encounter with an uncohesive, volatile group whose members reacted to self-revelation and emotional closeness with avoidance and anxiety reactions.

Planful Avoidance of Direct Questioning

These youngsters apparently perceived direct questioning and information-seeking, by the therapist, as an attack and a demand that they feed him. For a person schooled in the usual modes of conducting psychotherapeutic session, this was most difficult. It is significant that in an earlier stage of the group when the therapist was actively questioning and seeking information as to their lives and activities, they frequently caricatured him in their drawings, as a bizarre and menacing creature with bulging X-ray eyes. At times, their discomfort with this was more bluntly expressed as when one boy threatened, "I'm going to shoot you or cut your throat, you ask too many questions!" There was so much fear of and resistance to direct questioning that we refrained from this.

At times the therapist dealt with resistance phenomena by assuming responsibility for it with his own ego rather than directly or subtly charging group members with their behavior or demanding more mature behavior from them. This approach was based on our attempts to estimate the developmental level of the group at any given time and to gear our therapeutic efforts to that stage. When the group was perceived as being on the oral level, preoccupied with its own hunger for basic gratification, this obviously was not the appropriate time for confronting it with demands for behavior consistent with higher levels of maturation which the group members had not yet attained. At a later point when the members' capacity to assimilate frustration had been strengthened, group resistances could be brought more directly to their attention. Thus, at a particularly resistant point where there was a marked drop in attendance, the therapist said, "I have the impression I've been making the group uncomfortable. What have I done to make this place so awful; could you guys help me understand this?"

We also came to learn that protection of individual members' ego and reduction of threat could be enhanced by asking the group about an individual's behavior rather than asking the member himself, i.e. "Why is James so quiet today"? rather than "James, why are you so quiet?" Thus, object-oriented rather than ego-oriented questions were therapeutically preferable and more effective.

Respecting their Right to Distrust

Based on the recognition that the group members' distrust served a vitally needed defensive function against dangerous closeness, the therapist supported their right to be distrustful. In one of the beginning sessions, in response to group suspicion, the therapist commented, "It seems no one in this group trusts anyone else, including myself. Maybe you're smart not to trust me." This led directly to their proclaiming their quite limited trust of the therapist which then led in turn into an open expression of distrust of their mothers. "My mother would turn me in to the cops; she wants to kick me out of the house; she doesn't care if I die or not; you know when I was born my mother wanted to leave me in a garbage can near the hospital." In other words, the difficulty of our therapeutic task was compounded by the fact that we had to simply <u>accept, and at time even support as part of our operating framework</u>, a basic distrust of us.

Facilitating the Verbal Expression of Hostility and Allowing Primitive Fantasies to Emerge

The therapist's acceptance of the group members' distrust of him and of their hostile and aggressive fantasies resulted in increased verbal expression of such feelings. A dynamic theme of hostility and revenge emerged toward the deserting, ungiving and potentially dangerous father. After a particularly violent verbal barrage directed toward the therapist, one youngster said, "It's a good thing you have a short temper, I mean a long temper. You're probably saying to yourself, 'If you were my son I'd break every bone in your body'." Another youngster said, "If I grabbed the cake at home like this they'd cut off my hands and fingers." In one session the boys talked about how they would react if they met their real fathers again. One boy said, "If I met my father in the street, I'd beat him up." Another said, "I won't meet mine, he's dead." A third boy commented, "I'd ask him for money."

On several occasions when the therapist, to a limited degree, planfully took on some of the aspects of the "bad father," the members were then able to further express their feelings toward their own fathers. On one occasion when the therapist planfully frustrated the group's wish for Christmas presents, Steve said, "You're cheap, just like my father, you're a no-good nigger, you probably wouldn't give me anything if you were my father. I'd kill you off when you're 65."

The tension alleviated through the expression of their primitive, hostile feelings and fantasies, gradually made room for more direct expression of deeper and more stringently defended dependency longings. Perceptions of how unwanted they were by their parents emerged. One boy asked why he was the oldest in the group and in every group he had been in. "I don't want to be the oldest, I want to be young, I wish I was born old and got younger all the time." He then added that the unhappiest day of his life was the day he was born. Another youngster commented to this, "No, it was your mother's unhappiest day, not yours."

There is a good deal of discussion in the field about the wisdom of allowing patients like these to express primitive fantasies, rather than help them in repressing them. However, we found that these youngsters were so preoccupied with these fantasies that trying to help them repress them was virtually impossible. In addition, fostering repression would have alienated them further from the therapist, since this would have implied a rejection and denial of one of their main concerns, and would have indicated to them that their impulses and fantasies had the actual and feared reality value.

A somewhat puzzling aspect of this group was the almost complete absence of sexuality from their verbal productions; nor was there evidence of the pseudo-sexuality that one often sees in young adolescent groups before underlying feeling levels are reached. This appeared to be related to the group's compelling need, when given the opportunity, to express deprivation and frustration, aggression and their apparent perception of the therapist, for most of the life of the group, as the preoedipal mother. One may speculate whether and in which form sexuality would have emerged had the group continued into a third or fourth year when competitive feelings toward the therapist as a male might have replaced the earlier maternal transference.

Conclusions

Beginning tentatively and experimentally, we gradually evolved modified technique for approaching and treating a group of delinquent boys. We found, in working with them, that we could not effect them through the usual therapeutic group techniques and that any modicum of success depended upon our acceptance of and respect for their suspicious and mistrustful assumptions about life and other people. Our approach, pace and intensity was geared to this. Modified technique included: use of food, spontaneous expression of the therapist's own feelings and an analysis of them; the avoidance of direct questioning; respecting the boys' right to distrust; and encouraging verbal expression of hostility.

The feelings induced in the group therapist--the counter-transference--provided a valuable aid in achieving an emotional understanding of the group members' life experiences. This use of induced feelings also helped the therapist to develop a degree of emotional insulation needed to withstand the emotional onslaught to which he was exposed. These modified techniques enabled the group to function for two years. There was a shift in the extent of delinquent anti-social behavior and some obvious changes of functioning in the group, as the group members were able to move from motoric to verbal expression. We learned that these children could be reached in interview group therapy provided that the therapist is willing to listen and to change. However we did not know if these gains were sustained since there was no follow up.

Notes and Bibliography

1. Aichhorn, August, Wayward Youth. New York: Viking Press, 1935.
2. Bowlby, J., "Maternal care and mental health." Geneva World Health Organization Monograph. 1957.
3. Cohen, Albert K. Delinquent Boys: The Culture of the Gang. Glencoe, Ill.: Free Press, 1955.
4. Epstein, N. & Slavson, S. R., "Further observations in group Psychotherapy with adolescent delinquent boys in residential treatment." International Journal of Group Psychotherapy. Vol. 12, No. 2. 1962.
5. Freud, Anna, "Adolescence." Psychoanalytic Study of the Child. Vol. XIII, International University Press, 1958, p. 255-278.
6. Freud, Sigmund, Group Psychology and Analysis of the Ego. Standard Edition, 18, 1921.
7. Miller, Walter B., "Focal Concerns of Lower-Class Culture." Journal of Social Issues, Vol. 14, 1958, p. 5-19.
8. Rosenthal, Leslie, "A Study of Resistance in a Member of a Therapy Group." International Journal of Group Psychotherapy. Vol. 13, No. 3, 1963.

9. Slavson, S. R., Analytic Group Psychotherapy. New York: Columbia University Press, 1950.

10. Slavson, S. R., "Para-analytic Group Psychotherapy: A Treatment of Choice for Adolescents." Acta Psychother, Psychosom., Vol. 13:32, 1963.

11. Spotnitz, Hyman, "The Borderline Schirophrenic in Group Psychotherapy." International Journal of Group Psychotherapy, Vol. VII, No. 2. 1957.

Part II

Diagnosis and Treatment of Parents

10. Going Along with Defenses in Resistive Families

by Sidney Love and Herta Mayer

From *Social Casework*, February 1959.
Reprinted by permission.

Many parents apply for help to agencies providing child guidance services after they have been put under considerable pressure to do so by school and court authorities. In their initial interviews, these parents often defiantly deny their quite obvious need for help. They may state that their child has improved so much since the time of the court or school referral that they no longer see the need for service. If there has been a threat of expelling the child from school, the parents may angrily place the blame for the difficulties on poor school facilities and inadequate teaching methods. Stressing that neither they nor their child are "crazy" or in need of therapy, they often maintain that a change of school will provide a solution to the problem.

It is generally recognized in social work that much remains to be learned about effective methods of working with resistive families. The Youth Board study, *How They Were Reached*, is an example of the effort on the part of casework practitioners to gain better understanding of the reluctance of certain families to utilize necessary help. "The techniques most effective for serving these [resistive] families are still in process of evaluation and development, but the findings of this study indicate that they can be developed and that some of the community's most troubled children can be helped."[1] Another report also throws light on the clinical problem: "Frequently, the child with acting-out problems is brought to treatment only after a series of pressures from neighbors, teachers and often the law. . . . Implicit in these situations is the fact that motivation for treatment is often superficial and ambivalent. Obviously a parent who receives gratification, albeit unconscious, is not anxious to remove his source of supply, and a child attempting to satisfy parental wishes is not driven to seek help which will separate him from a needed parent."[2]

In this paper we shall present some theory and case illustrations that indicate why and how resistive parents may more readily respond to treatment if the worker understands their defenses and, in the early contacts, goes along with the defenses.

Understanding the Parents' Defense

When parents say that their child does not need treatment, when he obviously does, what is the emotional meaning of this defensive attitude? Otto Fenichel states: "Ego defenses may be divided into (a) successful defenses which bring about a cessation of that which is warded off, and (b) unsuccessful defenses which necessitate a repetition or perpetuation of the warding off process to prevent the eruption of the warded-off impulses . . . . All pathogenic defenses have their roots in childhood . . . ."[3]

In an article dealing with parental feelings in relation to their disturbed children, Yonata Feldman says: "[In some individuals their] early primitive strivings are kept in check only with the greatest expenditure of energy-- . . . sometimes through isolation and withdrawal. Somehow they are able to manage through part of their lives. Often the routine of a job makes their existence possible and checks anxiety from becoming overwhelming. However, when these individuals marry and have children, their problems are recreated. The normal developmental stages of the infant and growing child reactivates in them the same state of anxiety they had at this stage of their own development. Driven by anxiety, they may become extremely punitive to the child for fear that the child will not be able successfully to outgrow this particular stage of development which they themselves were unable to master. Or else, in fear of their own aggressive or seductive wishes, and to protect the child, they withdraw from the child emotionally . . . . Thus it is that the parent's anxiety in reaction to a certain developmental stage in the child overstimulates or understimulates the child and produces the same problem in the child as the parent had--often in a much more exaggerated form."[4] In another study of antisocial acting out of children, Hyman Lippman reports: " . . . in many instances the neurotic acting out of the child is nurtured by unconscious conflicts in the parents, particularly the mother. These neurotic mothers unable to act out their own hostile aggressive behavior, found it possible to get some gratification for their poorly repressed drives through unconsciously permitting their children to behave as they would have liked to behave."[5]

In the cases we studied, we found that the fundamental difficulty of these parents was their inability to deal with their impulses. Instead of verbally expressing their problems and conflicts, they seem impelled to demonstrate them in the form of avoiding treatment. Their resistiveness appears to be a sort of language, a primitive way of expressing opposition to authority. In waiting to be forced by public authorities to seek help for their children, these parents may be symbolically repeating their reactions to discipline situations of childhood when they experienced a high degree of pressure from persons in their environment. It is characteristic of persons who have suffered trauma of this nature that such behavior must be repeated. Now, as adults, and especially as parents, they must repeat their opposition to outside insistence that they or their children need help. The antisocial behavior of their children provokes the authorities to force them to go for treatment, and, being forced, they are roused to feelings of inadequacy and resentment.

Unable to express such feelings directly to the threatening authority figure, they often verbally submit to the referral but later rebel against utilizing the help offered by the agency. Their pattern of displacing anger is not only a repetition of their relationship to their parents, but it is often present in their child's conduct disturbance. From the viewpoint of reality, resistive parents have problems, but they also have an emotional need not to see, feel, or verbalize them. As rational adults, they should be able to admit that there is something wrong with them or their children. Emotionally, however, they react, when the caseworker confronts them with the seriousness of the situation, as if they are being criticized; or they may become suspicious of the worker, viewing him as an ally of a strange and hostile world. As a result, they tend to break off contact and, if pressed, become even more reluctant to discuss their problems since nothing has been offered to reduce their defiance.

At the point of the initial contact, we usually do not have sufficient information to make a definitive differential diagnosis. Nor do we have sufficient developmental data to understand fully the origin or the depth of the resistive pattern. We know, however, that reactive conduct disorders often have their roots in traumas experienced during the discipline (anal) stage of psychosexual development. Freud states: "The process of defecation affords the first occasion in which the child must decide between a narcissistic and an object-loving attitude. He either parts obediently with his feces, offers them up to his love or else retains them for the purposes of auto-erotic gratification; and later as a means of asserting his own will. The latter choice constitutes the development of defiance, a quality which springs therefore from a narcissistic clinging to the pleasure of anal erotism."[6]

On the basis of such clinical understanding and on our experience in practice, we have hypothesized that resistive parents did not receive the necessary parental protection in childhood which would have permitted them to integrate in a mature and harmonious way their infantile strivings with the adult side of their personalities. Lacking this protection in their developmental years, they subsequently have tried to find their own salvation by use of substitute defensive processes. Although they remain emotionally incapable of adequately fulfilling their parental role, they are compelled to present themselves as capable and self-sufficient parents. In this way, they deny the "child" in themselves as well as their dependence upon outside figures. Their need for case and protection continues, however, and they are not able to acknowledge their helplessness until their sense of a "weak world" has been strengthened. They can achieve a feeling of strength if the worker supports their defenses in the early contacts and does not attempt to attack them prematurely. We can say that resistive parents need their defenses, which is another way of saying that they require psychological protection in the casework contact. Such protection is provided them when the worker understands where they stand emotionally; that is, they are responding as children who have suffered traumas of the pre-oedipal stages of development.

The Role of the Caseworker

In studying our cases, we tried to understand our own emotional blocks that prevent us from going along with our clients' defenses. A familiar casework principle is that we start where the client is and that we do not move faster than he is ready to go. It is usually not difficult to follow this principle, provided our clients are willing to come to the agency and to give us the feeling that our help is needed. Once the worker feels that his help is accepted, he usually is able to respond to his clients in an emotionally appropriate manner. With resistive clients, however, the worker often finds it difficult to perceive how they are responding to him. When they deny a need for treatment and break appointments, the social worker, traditionally attuned to an actively giving role, tends to feel rebuffed. Feeling rejected, he may then be impelled to point out how much his help is really needed. The clients, in turn, will feel that they are not understood, with the result that they often abandon treatment.

It is important to remember that, emotionally, resistive parents recoil from reality. They may exonerate themselves and blame the environment, but when they do they have an overpowering need to use such defenses. It therefore seems imperative, in the initial stage of contact, for the worker to join with them in their stubborn denial that something is wrong with them or their children. If the worker understands the defense and the parents' unconscious communications, he then will not try to enlist the co-operation of an adult ego, which in fact does not exist. He will not burden these clients with early interpretations, nor will he present the reality situation to them as long as they are not ready to look at it. Rather, he will ally himself with them psychologically, looking at the world from their viewpoint and speaking their symbolic language. Thus, they may be able to verbalize hostile and dependent feelings and to modify their defiant attitude. They may then voluntarily involve themselves and their children in further treatment.

Case Illustrations

In order to show the application of these principles

in intake, two case illustrations will be presented. In both instances, the caseworker first endeavored to establish contact by going against the client's defensive denial of the need for help. Subsequently, the worker changed the approach, going along with the client's defense, which resulted in marked changes in the client's attitude toward utilizing the services of the agency.

First Approach--Going against the Defenses: Joel P, a 13-year-old boy, came to the attention of the court when he tried to burglarize a store. In court, Mr. and Mrs. P denied that Joel was in need of help, but claimed that he was a well-behaved child who had got into bad company and had been misled by other boys. They were certain that he would never repeat such an act again. The court made a referral to the agency.

The intake worker received the court report and, when he did not hear from the parents for several weeks, he telephoned Mrs. P. Mrs. P gave many reasons why she was not able to come to the office. The worker insisted repeatedly that it was necessary for Mrs. P to be seen in order to discuss Joel's problems. Finally, after much persuasion, Mrs. P agreed to send her husband. The worker accepted her suggestion and immediately sent Mr. P an appointment letter.

In his interview, Mr. P tried to minimize his son's difficulties. He said he was certain that his son knew now that he had done something wrong and said Joel had promised not to repeat such behavior. Mr. P felt, therefore, that there was no need for the agency's help. He blamed the neighborhood and spoke with tense hostility about the probation officer who looked upon him as if he were a murderer. The worker merely listened to this attack, but he still insisted that Joel needed help.

Further scheduled appointments with Mr. P were not kept. After additional pressure, Mr. P agreed to a second appointment. In this interview, he expressed stronger hostility toward the probation officer. He also spoke of Joel's improvement. The worker questioned the stability of this improvement and pointed out that the boy might become a delinquent. The father reluctantly permitted Joel to come in once to the agency, but then telephoned to inform the worker that the parents had consulted their family physician, who had advised them to leave Joel alone, and that coming to the agency would only make him more nervous.

Second Approach--Going with the Defenses. In the meantime, the caseworker had recognized that he had put too much pressure on Mr. and Mrs. P and had perhaps made them more resistive. He therefore now went along with their suggestion to discontinue at this point, especially if they thought this was a place that made people more nervous. He, however, offered them the agency's help whenever they might wish to return.

About eight months later, Mrs. P called the worker and immediately referred to his remark that "they could always come back." Mrs. P stated that she had many difficulties. Her husband had had an accident at work, had been hospitalized, and was now unemployed. In the interview which followed, Mrs. P mentioned the adverse effects that all these difficulties had had on Joel. However, when the worker tried to explore Joel's problems, Mrs. P was evasive and spoke immediately of the child's remarkable improvement. The worker, in contrast to his previous approach, did not question Joel's improvement. Instead, he asked whether any help was really necessary since Joel had already improved. The worker also pointed out, using Mrs. P's own previous statement, that taking care of the children and her husband was an exacting job and coming here might only add another burden. Mrs. P now insisted that she could find the time and that everything was not going as smoothly as she would like. When the worker wondered whether Joel himself was ready to come, Mrs. P said, with a smile, that actually he always had been willing to come, but that the parents were the ones who had been against it. The worker advised her to think over the idea of treatment. The following day Mrs. P called and stated definitely that both she and Mr. P wanted help.

How can we explain Mrs. P's change in attitude? In the first contact, she had not requested treatment. When the worker did not minimize Joel's difficulties, as the mother did, Mrs. P withdrew from contact and pushed the responsibility onto her husband. Mr. P seemingly came under threat, and the situation forced him to admit his failure as a parent and as an individual. As the worker insisted on Joel's need for help, Mr. P became more reluctant to acknowledge that there might be something wrong with his son. He also became more hostile toward the probation officer; that is, he indirectly expressed his anger at the worker who, he felt, had not treated him with respect and had criticized him unjustifiably.

The worker had prematurely treated these parents as adults, expecting them to cooperate with the agency. He had thought that they would be able to estimate realistically, just as he and the court had done, their need for help. Both parents, however, were emotionally unable to admit or reveal their feelings about themselves. Mrs. P could not acknowledge that she felt inadequate as a mother because she herself had craved care and attention as a child; and Mr. P could not reveal his irrational need to discharge destructive impulses through his son.

After the worker gained increased understanding of the defenses of both Mr. and Mrs. P, he had the opportunity to reverse his approach. In the second contact, he did not expose the parents to a possible narcissistic injury but, instead, went along with their initial defense--that they were adequate people and not in need of help. With this support, Mr. and Mrs. P both felt safe enough to disclose additional difficulties and to ask for the agency's service.

<u>First Approach</u>--Going against the Defenses: A school principal telephoned to refer Mark, age 10. He described the boy as disruptive and immature. A letter was sent to his mother requesting that she telephone our agency on a certain day. Mrs. B did not call until five days later. She stated that the principal had threatened to expel her son from school unless she went for treatment. She said that recently her boy had quieted down considerably in school. She agreed reluctantly to come to the office for a consultation, but she broke the appointment. Several attempts were made during the next month to arrange an office interview, in which the worker continued to put pressure on Mrs. B. She finally kept an appointment.

<u>Second Approach</u>--Going with the Defenses: Mrs. B began the interview by asking angrily, "What have you to tell me?" The worker responded by asking what Mrs. B wished to tell the worker. Mrs. B answered: "My son is not a psychiatric problem." She continued to talk, saying

that Mark's difficulties in school were due to poor teaching methods, to overcrowded schools, and to other disturbed children. The only reason she came to the agency was because the principal had threatened to expel Mark. The worker then said that many teachers used poor methods, that schools were overcrowded, and it was undesirable for anyone to be forced to go to an agency for help, particularly for help that a child might not need. Mrs. B responded by expressing intense resentment against the principal. She said she hated to be forced and that she had wanted to "tell the principal off." He made her feel as if she were "crazy." At this point, she said that she knew very well that she and her boy needed help. She explained that she had nervous indigestion; she had been examined for gallstones, but no physical basis for her gastric upsets was found.

She spontaneously recalled that she had had similar trouble with school authorities when she was a child; she always disobeyed teachers. She went on to say that she was not the kind of person who can easily ask for help. She said her mother had been seriously ill recently. Her father could cry. She always had to appear as the strong one. She wished she could change and learn to cry. If she could cry, she would feel great relief. She began to sob in the interview.

She also said that she had met some helpful psychiatrists in the hospital where she worked as a clerk and she had learned from them that you need not be crazy to go for therapy. She would very much like to have help for herself and her boy.

Mrs. B's initial rejection of treatment for her son seemed to be connected with her fear of her own infantile impulses, which she equated with mental illness. Her intense resistance to treatment reversed itself when she sensed that the worker understood her need to deny her son's obvious difficulties. The worker's verbal support of her defense of denial and projection enabled her to ventilate her feelings of resentment toward the threatening principal. Following this healthy discharge of feelings, she recalled her own school difficulties as a child. She then revealed a digestive symptom and expressed a desire to change her personality, "to learn to cry for help," and was able to request necessary treatment for herself and her son.

Summary

Some parents, who are placed under pressure by outside authorities to seek treatment for their children's conduct disorders, may, in intake, reveal their own pathogenic defenses by denying the need for help. Social workers often tend to point out to the parents the child's problems and the need for treatment. However, the parents then feel attacked and criticized, and may subsequently break off treatment. We have found that these parents do respond to offers of help if the worker first understands their unconscious language expressed in their resistance. By responding with similar language, the worker can often enable them to verbalize hostile and dependent feelings and to recall spontaneous memories of their own childhood deprivations and disturbances. Having attained some catharsis and beginnings of self-insight, these once hard-to-reach parents then become mobilized to ask voluntarily for treatment for themselves and their children.

Notes

1. How They Were Reached, Monograph No. 2, New York City Youth Board, New York, 1954, p. 90.
2. Mary E. Giffin, M.D., Adelaide M. Johnson, M.D., Edward Litin, M.D., "Specific Factors Determining Antisocial Acting Out," Amer. J. Orthopsych., Vol. XXIV, No. 4 (1954), p. 676-677.
3. Otto Fenichel, M.D., The Psychoanalytic Theory of Neurosis, W. W. Norton & Company, New York, 1945, p. 141, 143.
4. Yonata Feldman, "A Casework Approach Toward Understanding Parents of Emotionally Disturbed Children," Social Work, Vol. III, No. 3 (1958), p. 26.
5. Hyman S. Lippman, M.D., "Introductory Remarks," "Symposium, 1954-Antisocial Acting Out," Amer. J. Orthopsych., Vol. XXIV, No. 4 (1954), p. 667.
6. Sigmund Freud, "On the Transformation of Instincts, with Special Reference to Anal Erotism," Collected Papers, Vol. II, International Psycho-Analytic Library, Hogarth Press, London, 1949, p. 168.

11. Casework with Ego-fragmented Parents

by Herbert S. Strean

From Social Casework, April 1968.
Reprinted by permission.

One of the axioms of casework theory is that parental influence on a child is exerted not only by what his parents say and do but also by the kind of persons they are--that their total behavior, both conscious and unconscious, has a profound impact on the child.[1] A child's pathological behavior is frequently stimulated by conflicts in his parents, who, unable to express or sublimate their impulses maturely, permit him to behave as they would have liked to behave.[2] Parents of acting-out children usually offer subtle rewards for their behavior, whereas parents of neurotically inhibited children characteristically prevent acting-out by withdrawal of friendliness and other forms of positive recognition except on those occasions when the child inhibits himself or submits to parental dictates. The child, consequently, becomes unwilling to relinquish neurotic or acting-out pleasures because he is so frequently the recipient of love premiums when he demonstrates his sensitivity and acquiescence to parental desires.[3]

As Yonata Feldman has stated, if we acknowledge that the parent-child relationship is a crucial factor in a child's emotional development and that emotional disturbance in a child frequently justifies the assumption that his parent is either presently disturbed or was as a child, it follows that a parent's capacity to serve as a helpful model for identification has been impaired by his experiences with his own parents.[4] Unprepared for emotionally healthy living because he was improperly nurtured, the parent maintains a relationship with his child that is dynamically similar to the one he experienced in his own childhood. A state of anxiety is activated in the parent that corresponds to his state of anxiety in a similar state in his early psychosocial development.

Most practitioners working in the area of parent-child relationships are now intensely aware that when a parent describes a child's manifest problem, he simultaneously expresses and describes lacunae in his own emotional development. References to a child's sexual confusion, for example, are often the parent's means of requesting sexual information and guidance for himself as well as help for the child. Similarly, a child's school phobia is usually a reflection and manifestation of the parent's own separation anxiety; a parent's statement that his child does not respond to limits is frequently a disguised cry for aid in coping with his own aggressive impulses.[5]

The caseworker, therefore, faces the impact of a whole range of human feeling as he meets a parent in treatment. Not only is the parent reporting vignettes of his child's life circumstances; he is also exposing certain facets of his own life style in these reports.[6] As a parent describes his child's defective ego-functioning, it may be tentatively inferred that he is also pointing to gaps in his own ego apparatus. He asks the caseworker to provide the necessary resources to cope with the child's difficulties because he, the parent, feels very limited, if not impoverished.

The Ego-fragmented Parent

Despite a diverse array of sound treatment procedures to help parents modify disturbed relationships with their children, there is a kind of parent who frequently confounds the best-intentioned and most highly skilled worker--the ego-fragmented parent. Frequently such a mother or father comes to an agency involuntarily and is antagonistic toward the referral source and the agency as well. He views the school, the neighborhood, and other community institutions as precipitating, if not directly causing, his child's problems. Or he may ascribe the source to his spouse, his mother-in-law, or the child's older sibling. On occasion, the child himself is described as the one who is at fault: "There is a core of meanness in him, and no matter what I say, he just has to defeat me." The caseworker is often appealed to plaintively: "I know I do everything that a good parent is supposed to do, but he rebels and that's all there is to it."

The chief characteristic of such a parent is that his pathology manifests itself almost exclusively in his disturbed relationship with his child while many of his ego functions appear to be intact. He may be an effective employer or employee, and even a sensitive and affectionate spouse; however, in his nurturing relationship with his youngster, anxiety abounds. In contrast to the ego-deficient client, who shows pervasive weaknesses in regard to many ego-functions and therefore has difficulty relating in most psycho-social situations, this parent responds appropriately to many stimuli except when his child is involved. Reminiscent of the client who functions reasonably well only until an encapsulated paranoid system becomes activated and then responds with delusions of reference and persecution, the ego-fragmented parent can appear logical, rational, and well integrated, and he can demonstrate appropriate insight, if his child is not the subject or object of his attention.

On examination it appears that the parent-child relationship is a part broken off or detached from the rest of this client's psychic apparatus, evidence of a fragmented ego. Although a calm leader in a committee meeting, this parent is explosive with his son on the baseball field, often cursing him in front of his playmates because the boy did not slide into second base with appropriate athletic prowess. A sociable friend and affable bridge partner, such a person rages at the slightest provocation at a PTA meeting, seriously distorting others' remarks and bellowing unfinished sentences. Succinctly, he _appears_ to function well, to have mature object relations, and to test reality adequately--but when his child is the subject or object of his attention cathexis, he appears to be borderline psychotic or to have a severe character disorder. At such times he resorts to primitive defense mechanisms, distorts reality, feels persecuted, and attacks almost anyone, including his child.

In contrast to the ego-depleted client, whose ego dysfunction is gross and consistent in most relationships, the ego-fragmented parent can whip his child mercilessly or quarrel with a pediatrician vehemently and a few minutes later emerge as a skillful leader in a business, political, or social meeting. In the context of this parent's general behavior, his behavior in relation to his child appears to be "out of character"; in reality it is a severe, encapsulated symptom in the form of immature behavior as a _parent_.

Resistance to Treatment

In a casework contact the recurrent theme in all these parents' presentations is that virtually everybody but themselves is activating the child's problem. Against attempts on a worker's part to focus on the parent's own anxiety, anger, or helplessness, he vigorously defends himself by denial, further displacement, and projection. When a worker offers supportive statements, the client distrusts his sympathy and empathy and not infrequently manifests paranoid defenses. A typical reaction is to question the worker's motive, usually in a most provocative manner and one designed to put the worker on the defensive. When the worker points out that he is merely interested in helping the client, the client frequently demonstrates his suspiciousness further.

A caseworker's attempts to offer concrete services as a means of stimulating a workable treatment relationship are also rejected, more often than not as being "humiliating" or "depreciating." Stereotypes of caseworkers as "do-gooders" and "Lady Bountifuls" are often invoked by these clients. Most of their responses to casework intervention are so negativistic that they inevitably induce negative reactions in a worker. When the worker points out that the client is attempting to forestall help and induce rejection, the parent usually experiences the interpretation as criticism and then counter-attacks. Such procedures as attempting to bring the client to reflect on his situation or review his past usually summon the most impenetrable defenses. Educational, or any, guidance is almost always rejected.

As the caseworker reviews some of these responses to professional help, he gradually concludes that his client demonstrates so much negativism, strong projection, and rejection of help because of an enormous feeling of threat when face to face with an adult who is in a position of authority. The worker soon realizes that he, the worker, is perceived as a force that threatens to disrupt a meaningful, albeit tenuous, balance--specifically, the balance of the parent-child relationship. It begins to be evident that a clarifying question or interpretation is experienced by the parent as a command to modify his relationship with his child, and to do so immediately. An analysis of his responses to any supportive or sustaining procedures demonstrates that he interprets them as attempts by the caseworker to seduce him into a different relationship with his youngster. Rigorously defending the psychological status quo, this client, when his relationship with his child is studied, often feels depleted, and his available energy is used defensively rather than psychosynthetically. When this child is discussed, he feels bombarded by anxiety and resorts to the use of such primitive defenses as projection and introjection.

Where the Client Is

It is of paramount importance that the caseworker interested in helping the ego-fragmented parent in his relationship with his child be able to understand how the client experiences and views the parent-child relationship. Because he is fixated at an early level of development, his child's movement up the psychosocial ladder threatens the very position he wants to preserve.

> Mrs. A, whose mother had been hospitalized when Mrs. A was a little more than one year of age, was advised to seek casework help by a physician because she was unable to wean her child from the breast. At first critical of the doctor who referred her and ascribing the weaning difficulty to her two-year-old daughter, Mrs. A, by the second interview, was championing the necessity of maintaining a symbiosis. "There is nothing more beautiful than nursing and I will not let you or anybody else break us up," she stated with strong conviction.
>
> Mr. B consulted his plant physician about his three-year-old son, who was constantly constipated and untrained for bowel and urine control. Mr. B insisted on examining the boy's feces almost daily. He discussed the issue with his son continually and found himself very preoccupied with the topic. When the intake worker asked Mr. B why defecating was of so much concern to him, he responded, "Why it gives me a feeling of importance. . . . I dread the day when I'll have to discuss sex, girls, and all that stuff with him. . . ."

It is clear from these illustrations that the parents vicariously enjoyed infantile pleasures and that the child was rewarded for maintaining a regressed position. The ego-fragmented parent, not out of malice, but out of anxiety, prohibits the further psychosocial growth of his child because the expression of drives to maturation would activate these same drives in him and produce unbearable anxiety. To this parent, his child is an alter ego--a narcissistic extension. The child is permitted what the parent permits himself or can vicariously enjoy; he is prohibited from doing or expressing what the parent's ego cannot tolerate.

On the rare occasion that an ego-fragmented parent applies voluntarily for casework assistance, it is usually because his child has either summoned enough courage, or has been stimulated by someone else, to move beyond the parent's parallel rung on the psychosocial ladder.

> Mr. C, who had a concealed but fundamental pattern of isolation and withdrawal, maintained a well-functioning schizoid type of existence. He had much pleasure in daily silent games of chess with his eight-year-old son. When his son was invited by a schoolmate to play chess, Mr. C experienced a sharp feeling of panic. He recognized that his acute migraine headaches had a psychosomatic basis and that he needed some kind of help. With some insight he asked the worker, "Do you think I'm so upset because my chess partner might really leave me and play chess with somebody else?"

Sometimes a spouse is viewed as the agent who is disrupting the homeostatic balance. And when the parent feels that the equilibrium of his relationship with his child is being threatened, his reaction to the disruption is sometimes acted out in his interaction with the offending spouse. When the client uses his casework sessions to heap abuse on, and ventilate his hostility toward, his marital partner, the threat to the child-parent symbiosis, which is precipitating the visit to the agency, is often overlooked by the worker.

> Mrs. D, a woman with much doubt about her own femininity, was able to find a husband who admired her assertiveness and aggressiveness. He never questioned her dominance or demeaning of him. When Tommy, the D's son, became six years of age and began to assert himself

> a little, Mrs. D became very critical of her husband. It took many months for the caseworker to realize that the cause of her behavior was her overwhelming anxiety because Tommy was behaving in a less passive manner. It eventually became clear that her increased onslaughts in the direction of her husband were displacements of anger that she really felt toward her son for daring to experiment with "being a little man."

A search for common characteristics in ego-fragmented parents must focus on an analysis of the ego, the psyche's most important agent for dealing with reality.[7] It becomes apparent that this parent has a developmental vacuum: with many of his infantile needs unfullfilled, this parent seeks to gratify them through his own child. Any sign of growth on the part of his child induces anxiety and terror with which his ego finds it extremely difficult to cope. Consequently, the parent strives to maintain the status quo in his relationship with his child through constricting the child's development.

Treatment Considerations

If one accepts the premise that ego-fragmentation is the central theme in the difficulties of the parents being discussed, it follows that techniques that foster further development of the ego should be utilized in casework treatment with them. However, as Hyman Grossbard has pointed out, techniques for fostering ego development are not so well formulated as techniques for reducing anxiety associated with neurotic symptoms. Historically, treatment techniques have evolved from work with neurotic patients and, as a result, have been designed to resolve ego-alien symptoms, reduce guilt, and relax repressive mechanisms. These techniques have been predicated on the presence of an ego with a reasonably good capacity for most object relations; fairly consistent reality-testing; and objective perception in most situations.[8] Though the neurotic person may feel immobilized, his defensive adaptation, in contrast to that of the ego-fragmented parent, can tolerate insight into his character patterns and salient relationships. Unlike the primitive defenses that are resorted to by the ego-fragmented parent under stress, the defenses of the neurotic client are frequently utilized to bring the worker closer to him, rather than to ward him off.

The principal difference between the treatment approach to the neurotic client and the treatment approach to the ego-fragmented client lies in the nature of the treatment relationship. With the former, the caseworker can work largely through the transference. With the latter, however, since he is lacking in capacity for object relations, a treatment relationship is not easily established. It is necessary, therefore, for the caseworker to create a situation that will stimulate the client's capacity to form an object relationship with him. The client must be provided with an experience with the worker that will enable him to cope with and possibly master the psychosocial and psychosexual learning problems of his early developmental years. The casework interviews must provide a "living rather than a reliving experience"[9] so that the client's developmental vacuum may be filled and maturational lags overcome.

Because the ego-fragmented parent has suffered enormous frustration at the hands of his parent and because he comes to the social agency manifesting difficulties in his role as a parent, it is incumbent on the caseworker to function *in loco parentis* to the client. As a good surrogate parent the caseworker attempts to ascertain the psychosocial and maturational needs of "his child." He ascertains whether his client needs help in resolving the nuclear conflict of trust versus mistrust or is still striving for the nurture of an omnipotent, omniscient parent from whom he cannot separate. The caseworker must consider whether his client needs to have limits established and a structure provided so that he can cope better with his drives. It is also possible that he needs sex education and guidance. Like a good parent, the worker attempts to provide the appropriate emotional nourishment for his psychological child, without contaminating their interaction with his own narcissistic wishes and unfullfilled desires. Focused on the developmental need of his client the caseworker offers appropriate doses of gratification, frustration, and education which appeal, not to the rational, intellectual processes of the mature adult ego, but to the primitive learning processes of the immature ego in the child.[10]

What does the surrogate parent in the form of a sensitive caseworker specifically do? He may feed "his child" psychologically if this is indicated; he may limit him; or he may join him in a light conversation--depending always on his assessment of the client's fixation point and developmental gap. Of paramount importance, the caseworker seeks to relate to that particular pathological part of the client that is interfering with his assuming a parental role with his own child--the fragment that is posing difficulties for both the parent and his child.

The worker takes his cue from what is presented as the child's problem--so frequently a manifestation of the parent's own distress. The worker then attempts to provide experiences for his client that the client has not received in sufficient abundance or with the appropriate lack of ambivalence from his own parents. Through a new experience with the caseworker, the parent may then recapitulate with his child the positive interaction that he has had in the treatment relationship, rather than the pathological one he has had with his own parents.

> Mrs. E was advised by the school psychologist to seek therapeutic help for her son, Jerry, who showed little spontaneity or warmth, seemed removed from teachers and peers, and was doing poor academic work. Mrs. E responded to the school psychologist's advice as if it were a court order and contacted a child guidance clinic immediately.
>
> In her intake interview, Mrs. E defended her son and attacked the school psychologist, the principal, and Jerry's teachers. After the worker acknowledged that academic people frequently do not understand psychological problems, Mrs. E attacked the caseworker who was interviewing her, the agency, and the "whole child guidance movement." She ended the interview before the appointed time and did not return to the agency for a month.
>
> On renewing her contact with the same worker, Mrs. E continued to denounce the agency and the school personnel, with whom she had become involved. She felt that she was being forced to come to the child guidance clinic; otherwise, she said, she would be "in trouble with the Board of Education." The worker stated firmly that if the Board of Education created

difficulties for her, he would intercede.

Less vituperatively but nevertheless sarcastically, Mrs. E commenced to "analyze" all professional social workers, psychologists, and teachers and stated that most of them were "neurotic and emotionally immature." The worker asked innocent and seemingly naïve questions about how social workers and other professional people "got that way." Mrs. E then discussed, with a certain amount of empathy, "the poor family background" of social workers, their "neurotic childhood," and their "poor childhood training."

Mrs. E spent several interviews assessing the personal dynamics of professional people, and especially social workers. When the caseworker again told Mrs. E that she was probably correct in most of her "diagnostic assessments," Mrs. E moved toward a discussion of her own family background. She described being "squelched" as a child, illustrating this theme with many concrete examples. She talked about being forced to satisfy her parents even though she realized that it was not for her own good. The worker offered a mildly sympathetic comment--that Mrs. E had had a rough time and seemed to have had almost no rights of her own. Mrs. E agreed, and two interviews later she initiated the discussion by remarking, "Jerry needs more independence. Can you help me with this?" When the worker explored her request further, asking her to tell him what kind of help she had in mind, Mrs. E said: "The kind of help where you'll continue to talk to me like you have been doing. You see, if I had different folks for parents, I'd be a different kind of mother and then Jerry would be different. If you keep on talking to me the way you have been doing, I'll feel better, and then I can make Jerry feel better."

Because Mrs. E was incapable of fulfilling her parental role maturely and because she saw Jerry as a narcissistic extension of herself, her aroused anxiety and distress had to be projected and displaced onto social workers, agencies, and school psychologists. To deny the infantile part of her own character structure and remain unaware of her symbiotic tie with Jerry, she presented herself <u>on the surface</u> as a self-sufficient person. Because Mrs. E so vigorously defended herself, the worker did not focus on Mrs. E's anger, her role in the relationship with her son, or her own history. Such intervention would have constituted for her a threat to her current psychic equilibrium. The caseworker, therefore, tried to protect Mrs. E's archaic defenses through not challenging her projections and displacements and, instead, supported them.[11] So the empathic worker speaks in the client's language, supporting defenses where they need support and joining resistances that need joining,[12] just as a sensitive parent makes a cooing response to his infant's coos.

As the caseworker enacted the role of a surrogate parent, ministering to the needs of "his preoedipal child," Mrs. E perceived him as a symbolic parent who sympathetically listened to her expressions of wishes and fantasies.[13] In contrast to Mrs. E's own parents, the worker did not attempt to outreason or "squelch" her. Inasmuch as Mrs. E could not cope with her son's developing assertiveness and aggression because her own parents had not allowed her sufficient expression of these impulses and drives, the caseworker helped Mrs. E express toward others the anger she harbored against her parents. By permitting strong expressions of anger and aggression toward himself, the agency, and other professional people and by reacting nondefensively and with interest, the worker helped Mrs. E move toward tolerating, with some composure, her son's growing assertiveness and his efforts to develop some measure of ego automony.

Summary

It is a truism that each parent, because of the unique story of his life, forms a unique relationship with his child. For the ego-fragmented parent who has strong resistance to change, whose ego functions as a parent are limited, whose psychic equilibrium depends on the maintenance of a delicate pathological parent-child relationship, and who has experienced severe deprivations in his own childhood, casework must focus on maturational needs. The worker, rather than furnishing understanding about psychic processes and interpersonal conflicts, attempts to provide emotionally corrective experiences within a remedial casework relationship. When an ego-fragmented parent is provided the appropriate emotional and psychological nourishment in his treatment experience, he may be able to modify his relationship with his child.

Notes

1. Yonata Feldman, "A Casework Approach Toward Understanding Parents of Emotionally Disturbed Children," _Social Work,_ Vol. III, July 1958, p. 23-29; Oscar Sternbach, "Arrested Ego Development and Its Treatment in Conduct Disorders and Neuroses of Childhood," _The Nervous Child,_ Vol. VI, July 1947, p. 306-17.
2. Sidney Love and Herta Mayer, "Going Along with Defenses in Resistive Families," _Social Casework,_ February 1959, Vol. XL, p. 69-74.
3. Sternbach, _op. cit._; Herbert Strean, "Treating Parents of Emotionally Disturbed Children Through Role Playing," _Psychoanalysis and the Psychoanalytic Review,_ Vol. XLVII, Spring 1960, p. 67-75.
4. Feldman, _op. cit._
5. Strean, _op. cit._
6. _Ibid._
7. Hyman Grossbard, "Ego Deficiency in Delinquents," in _New Approaches to the Treatment of Delinquency,_ Family Service Association of America, New York, 1962, p. 3-10.
8. _Ibid._
9. Hyman Grossbard, "Ego Deficiency in Delinquents," in _New Approaches to the Treatment of Delinquency,_ Family Service Association of America, New York, 1962, p. 8.
10. Marie L. Coleman and Benjamin Nelson, "Paradigmatic Psychotherapy in Borderline Treatment," _Psychoanalysis,_ Vol. V, Fall 1957, p. 28-44.

11. Herbert Strean, "Treating Parents of Emotionally Disturbed Children Through Role Playing," Psychoanalysis and the Psychoanalytic Review, Vol. XLVII, Spring 1960, p. 67-75.

12. Sidney Love and Herta Mayer, "Going Along with Defenses in Resistive Families," Social Casework, February 1959, Vol. XL, p. 69-74.

13. See Coleman, op. cit.

12. Treatment of Mothers and Sons in the Absence of the Father

by Herbert S. Strean

Reprinted with permission of the National Association of Social Work, from Social Work, vol. 6, no. 3, July 1961, p. 28-35.

The extensive impact of divorce and separation on the emotional life of a developing child is well known. The obstacles to be overcome and the burdens to be assimilated for the remaining parent and his child have been well described and documented in the literature.

In reviewing the studies on children who grow up without one parent, Neubauer found that most attention appears to have been devoted to the pre-oedipal period, particularly to the absence of mothering in the need-satisfying phase.[1] Investigations by Bowlby, Glaser, and Anna Freud "demonstrate the inexorability with which the infant requires instinctual satisfaction through one consistent empathetic mother, and how failing this through separation from the mother in the first year of life, his future may be threatened by vegetative dysfunction, disturbances in object relations and ego structure."[2]

While specific clinical studies describing the vicissitudes of treatment with fatherless children in general and the fatherless son in particular are sparse, the available material will bear brief review. In 1905 Freud, in his *Three Essays on the Theory of Sexuality,* reported the results of his investigations on patients with hysteria. He stated that "the early loss of one of their parents, whether by death, divorce, or separation, with the result that the remaining parent absorbs the whole of the child's love, determines the sex of the person who is later to be chosen as a sexual object and may thus open the way to permanent inversion."[3] In his study of Leonardo da Vinci, whose illegitimate birth deprived him of a father's influence until perhaps his fifth year and "left him open to the tender seductions of a mother whose only solace he was," Freud describes a type of male homosexuality in which etiological factors are the maternal seduction of a son because of the libidinal shift from husband to child and the absence of a paternal influence on oedipal development.[4]

Ferenczi in discussing the early histories of male homosexuals emphasizes a fixation on the lost father due to the absence of necessary and unavoidable conflicts between father and son.[5] Fenichel points to the reinforcement of the inverted oedipus complex in boys by the fantasy image of an absent father, and describes the guilt engendered by fantasy fulfillment of oedipal wishes when the same-sexed parent leaves the familial scene.[6]

Neubauer in his recent paper, "The One-Parent Child and His Oedipal Development," stresses the pathogenic potential of an absent parent and underlines the profound conflicts in sexual identification and superego formation found in the children he studied. While significant variables are seen--namely, the timing of the loss and the relationship of the child's sex to the sex of the missing parent--"the single parent's over-cathexis and consequent seduction of the child described by Freud may be considered prototypic." Further, "the fantasy objects of immensely idealized or sadistic dimensions which replace an absent parent are nearly ubiquitous."[7]

In "A Pattern of Mother-Son Relationship Involving the Absence of the Father," Wylie and Delgado of the Worcester Youth Guidance center comment that nearly all the twenty boys they investigated showed learning problems and had enormous difficulty handling their aggressive impulses.[8] The relationship between mother and son was described as "intense, highly sexualized, and full of hostility." The mothers had many conflicts about their roles as women and mothers and had conflicting attitudes toward men in general; their sons seemed to be used by them to solve these conflicts. Dominated by a "vengeful, competitive attitude toward males and by a strong wish to be a man, these women looked upon their sons as the fulfillment of this wish." The boy's role was that of the mother's dangerous, aggressive penis. The boys also represented the bad part of the mother which "must be displayed, fought and sometimes destroyed or confined." Wylie and Delgado reported that their attempts to help these patients were not very successful. Most of them either rejected treatment outright or withdrew after a few visits. Several factors which may have contributed to their poor therapeutic results are proposed. (1) These are often quite severely disturbed people, and to the degree of their pathology might be expected to limit therapeutic work. (2) Most of them were poorly motivated for therapy and came in at a time of crisis and under external pressures. (3) These women have great difficulty in giving up their sons, who serve as their sexual objects. The boys, too, struggle to maintain the situation and view the treatment as a threat to this source of pleassurable gratification.[9]

The dubious prognosis for the mother-son constellation described by Wylie and Delgado was reaffirmed by the child guidance personnel with whom they shared their findings at an Orthopsychiatric meeting in 1958. The consensus at this meeting was that, despite the well-intentioned efforts of many child guidance clinics and family agencies to involve this type of "broken" family in treatment, the results have not been proportionate to the therapeutic zeal invested. The mother, who frequently uses the son unconsciously as a psychological spouse, is most resistant to releasing him to another adult for treatment. "I want my son to myself, he is my whole life," is the message she seems to convey. She refuses to surrender her son to one person in the individual treatment relation, with its potential for exclusive possession, for it may stir up her own unresolved strivings and attachments to the most significant persons in her own life.[10] The son, although forced to fuse two objects into one, submits to his mother's wishes and resists therapy, as well. He supports the well-proven child guidance axiom that the child and his functioning are expressions of the parents' egos.[11]

Mother-Son Symbiosis

Our own experience in the Manhattan Office of the Madeleine Borg Child Guidance Institute seemed to coincide with those of others. Consequently we began to investigate intensively this type of family constellation and our therapeutic approaches to it. We can say upon review and reflection that the mother-child relationship appears to be a form of _folie à deux._ Just as "the paranoid develops for himself a partner, a paranoee, or an alcoholic man is married to a certain type of woman who will, against all expectations of her logically minded friends who want to save her, return to him and nurse him until he is strong enough to go on a drinking binge again,"[12] perhaps the mother unconsciously needs to provoke a similar situation with her son.

As the mother, in many cases, unconsciously sought a separation or divorce from her husband, does she not recapitulate this same phenomenon with her worker and want to divorce him as well? Further, as any human organism needs defenses for protection, may we not look at an emotional symbiosis as similar to a defensive layer of skin which, if pierced, will bleed? May not treatment symbolize for the mother and son we are studying a threat to their psychological equilibrium--the threat of disrupting a needed relationship? Upon careful scrutiny of our own reactions to these mothers, it seemed imperative to look upon them not as evildoers--which unfortunately we did at times--but as unhappy human beings caught in the net of their own frustrated wishes.[13]

As Feldman _et al._ in "A Casework Approach in Apparently Unreachable Cases" have pointed out,

> A fundamental problem in cases of extreme resistances is the difficulty of the client in dealing with his destructive and libidinal impulses and his need--instead of feeling and expressing them in language--to act them out--mainly in the form of resisting help. He has not received the necessary parental protection which would have allowed him to integrate his infantile strivings in a more mature way and in harmony with the more adult side of his personality. . . . Though he remains emotionally incapable of fulfilling his parental role, he is compelled to present himself as a capable, self-sufficient parent. In this way, he denies the "child" in himself, as well as the need for an outside protective figure.[14]

As Love and Mayer suggest, such protection becomes available when the worker places himself where the parent stands emotionally, namely, as a child. He does not try to enlist the cooperation of an adult ego which, in fact, does not exist. He does not ask for responsibility prematurely, he does not burden the client with early interpretations, and does not show the reality situation as long as the client is not able or does not wish to see it. He allies himself with the client psychologically, looks at the world from his viewpoint, speaks his language, and then can convey to him that it is not a sign of damage or inadequacy to seek infantile gratification and to continue the search for a healthy parent.[15]

One Therapist for Mother and Son

In formulating our hypothesis further, in order to support the defenses of the mother who wants "my son to myself" and of the child who attempts to satisfy his mother's wishes, we decided that to preserve rather than attack the symbiosis we would not "divide" the case. We felt it would be less threatening to the symbiosis for the mother to see the very person who treats her son. This enables her to have consistent access to this person, thus diminishing her fear that he will be alienated from her. Also, we speculated that if we offered the mother and son a male worker, would we not be reconstructing symbolically the family before it was disrupted? In a non-threatening relationship, could not the mother begin to invest some of her libidinal and aggressive drives in the therapeutic relationship instead of acting them out with her son? Would not the son gradually receive permission to enjoy a father figure if the mother could slowly transmit new heterosexual values to him?

These are the questions we asked. The following three cases will attempt to illustrate our experience within the framework of our conceptual thinking.

<u>Case 1.</u> Mrs. A, a middle-aged widow, divorced her husband when she was 35 years old. Although her marriage was always stormy, domestic harmony was completely unknown shortly after the birth of their son, which occurred three years after the A's were married.

Mrs. A was advised by her son's guidance counselor at school to seek therapeutic help for him. According to teachers' reports Robby, aged 13, appeared withdrawn, showed little spontaneity, spent much time immersed in fantasy talking to himself. His characteristic way of relating to peers was to be the "fall guy"; he submitted to their wishes when they suggested that he insult a teacher, lift a girl's skirt, or swear. Although the counselor suggested the idea of therapy as a possibility, Mrs. A responded to his proposal as if it were a court summons and called the clinic immediately.

In her initial interviews, Mrs. A was very quick to defend her son. "He has had a hard life and you can't expect too much from him. He has no father and I'm his whole life. I try my best and when he's lonely I get into bed with him and cheer him up. The people at the school are making a big mishmash out of this." When the worker agreed, saying that frequently school personnel do not understand well-meaning mothers who are very attentive to their sons, Mrs. A condemned the school for "making me think that my Robby is a problem." She damned guidance personnel and school personnel, and felt that "too much was made out of this psychiatry business. I can take care of Robby by myself. There are a lot of people who don't understand mothers and sons like me. I love my boy and nobody will take him away from me." When the worker stated that he couldn't think of anything much crueler than taking away Robby from his mother, Mrs. A remained silent for a few moments and then burst into tears. "People just don't understand. They don't understand," she sobbed. The worker said that he would like to understand.

Mrs. A went on for several sessions again damning educators, therapists, social workers, and others. When this was not challenged or interpreted, Mrs. A began to speak of her own history. "I've had to fight my way in life. Nobody cared about me. Nobody understood. My parents pushed me and I had to please them. I married the man they wanted, not who I wanted. I did everything for them." The worker took note of Mrs. A's experiences of being frequently squelched, ordered around, and defeated, and how this was being repeated with him. She responded during her fifteenth session, "Oh, I forgot to tell you. I let Robby join the Y on his own. I think it's good for him to do things on his own."

In subsequent interviews Mrs. A reported that Robby wanted to start seeing "that Strean guy." However, even when the worker repeated Mrs. A's previous doubts about psychotherapy, she said with conviction, "I am all for it, but Robby will decide for himself. I'll help him if he wants it."

This clinical illustration highlights some of the initial problems we have in treatment with the mothers under investigation. Incapable of fulfilling their parental roles appropriately and tending to see their sons as extensions of themselves, these mothers frequently project their inadequacies onto other people. To deny the infantile parts of their own characters and remain unaware of their symbiotic ties with their sons, they present themselves as self-sufficient people. As we observed in the case just described, the worker did not focus on Mrs. A's anger or her role in the parent-child relationship, for it would only have been perceived by her as a threat to disrupt her psychic equilibrium. Rather, he attempted to protect her archaic defense so that he could be perceived as a person who sympathetically listens to expressions of wishes and fantasies and does not attempt to interpret irrational ideas. As the worker also permitted Mrs. A's expressions of rage, and could slowly help her differentiate herself from her son, she was able to release some control over him and permit his entrance into the Y and eventually into treatment.

We learn from Mrs. A that through our protection of her defenses, her needed symbiosis, and her use of projection she could see us as an ally. However, despite our occasional successes in involving the mother in a relationship by offering her enough protection to enable her to release her son for treatment, we often observe rigid, seemingly impenetrable resistances erected by the son.

Case 2. Howie B, a 12-year-old boy, was referred for treatment by school personnel. Provocative and unruly in the classroom, he was failing most of his subjects despite a high I.Q. His peers frequently rejected him because of his clowning, baiting behavior. At home, he either watched television or talked to his mother about how his father "never gave me a break." Although the parents decided on a formal separation when Howie was 10 years old, prior to that there had been numerous separations and reconciliations.

As the displayed expression of family disturbance, Howie often carried out the unconscious mandate for instigating arguments and prided himself on his importance--"they fight over me."

Although Mrs. B was extremely resistive to receiving help for herself and Howie, after much support she was able to release him for treatment. In Howie's initial interviews he immediately attempted to involve the worker in arguments and fights. He made it clear that he had won an oedipal victory and that he could beat the worker very easily. "Look, Streanbones," he remarked during his sixth hour, "I've got your number! You think you can straighten me out? Well, you're mistaken! I've got a good deal all the way around and I don't care what the school says. I've got it made there, too. You can't win." Whereupon the worker casually remarked that Howie had been very capable in defeating his father, the school, and everybody else; it was a safe bet that even if the worker wanted to treat him, it was practically impossible. Howie laughed and said, "I guess you don't like to work too hard, huh?"

Since Howie's resistance to treatment was not attacked and the neurotic gratification he received not interpreted, the therapeutic encounter did not appear too forbidding to him. He could come for his sessions because "there was nothing else to do." But in interview after interview Howie attempted to provoke the worker in a truly creative manner. "I tell my mother what a jerk you are and she's beginning to agree . . . you're so dumb, you couldn't harm a flea, Streanbones." Session after session the therapist merely listened to Howie's remarks with mild interest and limited response. Occasionally he would say, "Oh, you can get rid of me any time. You did it with your own father," or "I'm sure you'll get your mother to fight with me. You are a master at that."

After seven months of coming to see the worker on a regular basis, Howie tried a new tactic. During one of the hours when Mrs. B was seeing the worker, Howie rapped on the door and demanded to see his mother immediately. While Mrs. B was ready to acquiesce, the worker sharply stated, "I am with your mother alone and we will not be interrupted or disturbed by you!" Mrs. B initially felt that the worker was being very cruel, but when he maintained a nondefensive attitude and attempted to explore her reaction, she began to recall how Howie would constantly interrupt her conversations with her husband and how he frequently entered the parents' bedroom, with no limits imposed on him. At the end of this hour Mrs. B declared, "You know, I can't exactly tell you why, but as I leave this office today I feel like a woman."

In Howie's next interview he yelled and screamed at the worker for not being able to share his mother with him for even a minute. "You want my mother all to yourself, don't you?" he belligerently queried. "At times I do," the worker replied. Though Howie spent several hours castigating the therapist for being so unfair, he finally modified his tone. "You're trying to be like an old man to me and show me that I'm a kid. You're a knucklehead but sometimes I see your point a bit."

As Mrs. B felt "more like a woman" with the worker and could put into words some of her libidinal and aggressive fantasies activated in the transference relationship, Howie could focus more on the gratification he received in "having my mother to myself and annoying you."

Although we have hypothesized that the mother and son, when seen by one worker and not divided, do not feel quite as threatened--and despite our belief that recapitulating the original family symbolically is, in a sense, gratifying to them--the parallel resistances of mother and son to relating to the male worker are none the less powerful. The following case illustration is typical in our experience. It highlights the similar resistances of mother and son.

Case 3. Mrs. C, an attractive woman of 46, had lived alone with her 14-year-old son Jimmy since he was 2 years old, when the parents divorced. She was referred to the clinic by her family physician when she discussed Jimmy's transvestitism with him. Jimmy, in addition, was doing poorly in his schoolwork.

Though both Mrs. C and Jimmy seemed eager for help, they quickly manifested strong resistances. Mrs. C complained bitterly about the fee, the appointment hour, the drabness of the office, the worker's poor choice of clothes, and his personal mannerisms. She felt that most men who enter the field of psychotherapy were probably homosexuals, and "anyway, how can a young kid like you help an experienced woman like me?"

Jimmy, too, didn't have much use for the worker. "I have gotten along without men all my life--who needs you?" He was quite sure that the worker had a concealed tape recorder and would use anything he discussed against him. Furthermore, he just didn't like school, and as far as his transvestitism was concerned, that was his business.

When the worker attempted to examine the fantasies ascribed to him without interpreting them and without counter-aggression, both mother and son felt that the worker had an "inferiority complex" and was too "insecure." When he showed interest, he was "overenthusiastic," and when he did not respond to their paranoid mechanisms he was experienced as cold, rejecting, and indifferent. After several months of these encounters the worker asked each of them what was going wrong. Most of his interventions seemed so unacceptable. To this Mrs. C replied by accusing the therapist of being too seductive and "trying to make" her, adding that "he certainly wasn't her type." She went on to relate that most men were no good--they had all disappointed her. Her grandfather, whom she truly loved, remarried after her grandmother's death and "this really hurt me." Her father was her mother's "puppy dog." "Mother's word was law and I got nothing. My husband was a 'shmoo,' and now most of my dates don't know which end is up. So you see, honey, you ain't got a chance."

Though Jimmy began to become interested in girls while his mother was focusing more meaningfully on the story of her heterosexual life, and although his schoolwork improved and his transvestitism diminished, as soon as the worker supported the C's temporary gains they both made strong bids to discontinue treatment altogether. Their wish to "go it <u>alone</u>--leave us <u>alone</u>" was ever present.[16]

Summary and Conclusions

Inasmuch as our study is till in its infancy, it is premature to state any definite conclusions. We are still involved in experimental investigation and need more clinical data and observations of others to support or refute our hypotheses.

While sufficient empirical data are lacking, we tend, after three years of study, to view the mother-son relationship under investigation as a powerful, albeit pathological, symbiosis. As a mutually gratifying network, neither mother nor son is eager for therapeutic assistance. They want to maintain the *status quo*, and when they do come for treatment it is usually under strong external pressure. The mothers have great difficulty in releasing their sons to another person because their psychological equilibrium, which is dependent on their sons, may be disrupted. The sons appear to be rewarded by their mothers for their unconscious sensitivity to their mothers' wishes, and they, too, resist therapy.

Looking upon these mothers not as evildoers but as human beings with conflicts is an often difficult but, of course, necessary attitude to maintain. Both mother and son must experience the worker not as an intruder who wishes to disrupt an emotional balance, but as a protector who seeks to help the mother and son preserve their relationship with each other. We have experienced a modicum of success when we have not "divided" the case but have centered the treatment of mother and son in one worker. If a part of the pair wishes to grow and enjoy family life, the provision of a male therapist helps them to re-establish a symbolic family. They are then able to modify to some extent their mutual need for and dependency upon each other.

The difficult but interesting mother-son constellation provides rich material for study and treatment, and challenges the therapeutic resources in us all.

Notes

1. P. Neubauer, "The One-Parent Child and His Oedipal Development," *Psychoanalytic Study of the Child*, Vol. 15 (New York: International Universities Press, 1960).

2. *Ibid.*, p. 287. *See also* J. Bowlby, *Maternal Care and Mental Health*, World Health Organization monograph (Geneva, 1951); K. Glazer and L. Eisenberg, "Maternal Deprivation," *Pediatrics*, Vol. 18, No. 2 (April 1955); and A. Freud, "Observations on Child Development," in *Psychoanalytic Study of the Child*, Vol. 6 (New York: International Universities Press, 1951).

3. S. Freud, *Three Essays on the Theory of Sexuality* (standard ed.; London: Hogarth Press, 1953), Vol. 7, p. 563.

4. *Ibid.*

5. S. Ferenczi, *The Nosology of Male Homosexuality: Sex in Psychoanalysis*, I. (New York: Basic Books, 1950).

6. O. Fenichel, *The Psychoanalytic Theory of Neurosis* (New York: W.W. Norton & Co., 1954).

7. Neubauer, *op. cit.*, p. 292.

8. H. Wylie and R. Delgado, "A Pattern of Mother-Son Relationship Involving the Absence of the Father," *American Journal of Orthopsychiatry*, Vol. 29, No. 3 (July 1959), p. 646-649.

9. *Ibid.*

10. L. Rosenthal *et al.*, "Family Relations as a Consideration in Selecting Children for Activity Group Therapy," *International Journal of Group Psychotherapy*, Vol. 10, No. 1 (January 1960), p. 79.

11. O. Sternbach, "Arrested Ego Development and Its Treatment in Conduct Disorders and Neuroses of Childhood," *The Nervous Child*, Vol. 6, No. 3 (July 1947), p. 307.

12. L. Knoepfmacher, "The Length of Treatment in a Child Guidance Clinic," *Jewish Social Service Quarterly*, Vol. 26, No. 2 (December 1949), p. 185.

13. L. Knoepfmacher, "Child Guidance Work Based on Psychoanalytic Concepts," *The Nervous Child*, Vol. 5 No. 2 (April 1946), p. 210.

14. Y. Feldman *et al.*, "A Casework Approach in Apparently Unreachable Cases," p. 11-13. Paper presented at a meeting of the American Orthopsychiatric Association, New York City, March 1958.

15. S. Love and H. Mayer, "Going Along with Defenses in Resistive Families," *Social Casework*, Vol. 40, No. 2 (February 1959).

16. H. Strean, "The Use of the Patient as Consultant," *Psychoanalysis and the Psychoanalytic Review*, Vol. 46, No. 2 (Summer 1959), p. 36-45.

13. On the Patient-Therapist Relationship In Some "Untreatable Cases"

by Oscar Sternbach and Leo Nagelberg

From Psychoanalysis, vol. 5, no. 3, Fall 1957. Reprinted by permission of The Psychoanalytic Review.

In 1955, The American Association of Psychiatric Clinics for Children sponsored a panel discussion on cases which, after years of treatment, are closed as "untreatable." Such cases are not at all rare: these children do not present special complications due to environmental factors, symptomatology encountered in them is not unusual, and they do not seem to require a special treatment method aside from the usual therapy provided by the clinic. Moreover, the mothers of these children are cooperative and continue treatment despite the fact that there has been little or no improvement even after years of therapy. Workers find it difficult to close such cases, and they are usually terminated only after long and painful conflict in the worker, frequently as a result of pressure by the agency.

A number of such cases, selected from the files of the Madeleine Borg Child Guidance Institute of the Jewish Board of Guardians, New York, were studied for this panel discussion and one of us (O. S.), presented the results of the study in a brief communication in which the following observations were made:

While there were personality differences in many respects in the mothers selected for the study, one could recognize in these cases an apparently typical constellation which would briefly be designated as a condition of 'repressed destructiveness.' The children in these cases were babyish, clinging and destructive. The mothers, while they did _act_ in a punitive fashion, never could _feel_ punitive or aggressive. They were mild-mannered, _polite_, were consciously willing to be helped and wanted to be told what to do or to be advised in an authoritative manner. In treatment they related in a compliant manner and their need for love and support seemed insatiable. However, a hidden competitiveness and hostility could be discerned beneath their demands for help which seemed to cloak a desire to defeat the worker. These mothers were rarely angry at the workers and, in fact, would praise them. They would present themselves as inadequate and worthless, accepting responsibility for the lack of improvement, but indirectly they seemed to accuse their workers of being inadequate since their failure in therapy was a reproach and living proof of the therapist's incompetence.

Conversely, the workers, although resentful and then guilty over their failure to improve these patients, responded to them in a friendly and most cooperative fashion, thus donning--in a replica of the behavior of the patient--the mask of kindliness to conceal, even to themselves, their own negative feelings and irritability.

Spurred on by the patient's helplessness, their childlike, and also flattering behavior, the worker would offer encouragement, guidance, support and numerous other gifts--including interpretations.

The worker's need to offer help became more urgent as the therapeutic failure became more evident. Though consciously of a most helpful disposition, the worker--with vision clouded in the counter-transference--would act in a non-curative fashion without realizing that feelings of resentment or personal drives of rivalry or domination were finding unconscious gratification in the fact that the case remained unimproved. In this way, beneath a pleasing and cooperative relationship, a mutually destructive struggle between patient and worker would lead to a defeat of treatment.

A closer study of this constellation led us to emphasize a specific defense against the underlying destructiveness in untreatable cases. This defense consists in feelings of weakness, inadequacy or worthlessness in these patients, and in an idealization of mother figures. The ego of these patients in regard to their own hate, their own destructive impulsivity is mute; and indeed we see that these patients hold parental figures, and later on, their workers, in the highest esteem.

Typically, our patients will describe themselves as mistreated, seeking the source of the difficulties in outside conditions, or, with a defense used in depressive reactions, will describe themselves as inadequate or worthless. The defenses may be formulated as follows: "I do not hate. I only hate if I have been mistreated" or "I do not hate anyone else, I only hate myself for being so inadequate."

The attitude of these patients toward parental figures may then be formulated somewhat like this: "I do not wish to destroy mother. I'm much too weak and helpless to even think of such a deed. All I want is help and love." These patients--as their history reveals, look upon their mothers as powerful, kind and perfect in an idealization which permits them to think of themselves, too, in an idealized way and which again protects them against feeling the hatred they have for themselves or for their parents.

One may now understand that this defense constellation, where a condition of helplessness and weakness has to be maintained at all costs, can present peculiar obstacles in the treatment relationship. To improve in therapy means to become less dependent, more competitive and more self-reliant. The understanding gained in therapy usually has the effect of strengthening the patient's ego, so that he can replace his primitive defenses with more socially acceptable ones. The usual therapeutic devices--represented roughly speaking, by non-censoring attitudes and by interpretations--far from strengthening the ego in our patients, may have the opposite effect.

Thus, if the therapist tries to explain directly to the patient that she is incorrect in blaming her environment but that she should look within herself and see in her own aggressions the source of her difficulty, the patient will feel blamed. Since she does not feel she is loved by the therapist who appears to her as critical, she will continue therapeutically in a refractory fashion, and is not willing to explore her own aggressive reactions. If the therapist refrains from all blame, sides with the patient, tries to remove anxiety and guilt feelings (necessary defenses against the underlying aggression), by falling in with the request of the patient and giving encouragement, advice or direction, then the therapist, since he is seen as too kind, may only increase feelings of worthlessness, with the result that the patient, even more unable now to feel and to deal with his underlying destructiveness, must continue in compliant and submissive ways.

Thus, if the therapist is kind and encouraging, the patient may feel encouraged to settle in a dependent role and also, in the face of so much kindness shown to him, may look upon himself as unworthy and will continue to see the therapist in an idealized light. If, on the other hand, the therapist is frustrating and, for instance, interprets the patient's behavior as aggressive or 'bad', this will increase the patient's anger, then lead to guilt and feelings of worthlessness. In short, no matter what the therapist does, his interventions will be responded to in a therapeutically negative fashion.

It seems that we deal here with the same therapeutic impasse which was described by Freud in The Ego and the Id as the so-called negative therapeutic reaction. Freud emphasizes that in these cases every therapeutic effort, every encouragement, every interpretation, which in other cases would lead to improvement, only cause stagnation or even an exacerbation of the illness. Freud traces the intractability of these cases to an extraordinarily strong unconscious guilt feeling, constituting a resistance which may be described by the formula, "I must not improve and be cured. I do not deserve it." Freud was rather pessimistic about the therapeutic outcome in these cases. While his assumption of a severe "unconscious feeling of guilt" as constituting an important factor in the barrier to therapeutic success can clinically be validated in our cases, our understanding of the defensive constellation in the so-called "untreatable" cases may warrant a brighter therapeutic outlook.

In addition to severe unconscious guilt feelings, we postulate a defense against the return of destructive impulses which, in spite of unusually strong resistances against becoming conscious, can be made available to the patient's awareness. This can be achieved by rather specialized treatment methods which make it possible for the patient to deal constructively with the underlying aggressive energy contained by the defensive structure.

We were fortunate enough to come across a case in which the patient showing all the characteristics of our "untreatable" cases as well as the "negative therapeutic reaction" described by Freud, began to relate more constructively in therapy as a result of a special treatment approach. This case was one among others in an experimental treatment project on "borderline" cases, carried out for a number of years at the Madeleine Borg Child Guidance Institute of the Jewish Board of Guardians, New York, under Dr. Hyman Spotnitz, by the staff of the Pronx office. In this case, treatment steps were taken which avoided the therapeutic dilemma mentioned and the patient's helplessness was changed into resourceful, constructive attitudes.

This was the case of Mrs. Y. and of her daughter Linda who, almost ten years old at the time of referral, wanted to be bottle-fed, would use abusive language or hit her own mother. Mrs. Y. remembered her own mother as a loving and most unselfish person, and similarly tried to be liked and approved by her worker who would maintain a friendly and encouraging attitude.

After a number of years of treatment, during which no appreciable improvement occurred and the patient continued to speak about her therapist in admiring terms, a change in the therapeutic climate took place when the worker finally realized that the suggestions she had been making at the patient's request were never carried out and were only used for defeatist purposes. The worker now began to withhold advice, study requests for help instead of satisfying them. The worker progressively imposed more and more frustration on the constant demands made by Mrs. Y. For instance, Mrs. Y. asked that her youngest daughter be taken into treatment; she was refused. For a number of years the family had managed not to pay the amount of fee they could afford. While they were able to take expensive trips, they refused to pay an adequate amount for the therapy. The worker now insisted that the family pay the higher fee which the family could well afford. Mrs. Y. began to feel that the worker--whom she had always regarded as a motherly person--turned out to be too interested in money or in "squeezing" her out.

Other similar types of frustrations released feelings of resentment against the worker. When Mrs. Y. once again complained about her husband, saying that he did not want to change, the worker said that he might indeed be incorrigible and how would it be were Mrs. Y. to leave her husband, perhaps even her children? Mrs. Y. was surprised at worker's attitude, which she thought was defeatist and cruel; then she tried to prove to the worker that her family situation did not require such drastic measures. She even told the worker of ways she could imagine to make her husband feel that he was "boss of the house." Mrs. Y. accused her therapist of being too pessimistic and thus became able to find solutions for problems which the worker appeared to consider insoluble.

Of course, Mrs. Y. often fell back into her hopeless attitude. She would continue to describe her struggles with her daughter, her helplessness to change the situation. The worker agreed that Mrs. Y. might possibly never be able to change the situation. This would prompt Mrs. Y. to prove that the worker was wrong and destructive in her attitude and that Mrs. Y. herself could handle the situation. On other occasions Mrs. Y. would say that her daughter was abnormal and beyond help. The worker now deliberately took the attitude that possibly the child could not be helped at all, might have to be given up as hopeless or perhaps even sent to a mental institution. Mrs. Y. became indignant and said she was going to prove that the child was normal in every way; she now proceeded to change her behavior toward her daughter, giving her greater freedom to grow in healthier ways.

Progressively, Mrs. Y. developed the feeling that she could figure things out, could solve problems as well as the worker and perhaps much better. Her worker was no longer the omnipotent mother whose constant care was needed. Whereas, in the preceding year she had continually defended her own mother as the perfect person, Mrs. Y. began to abandon this theme, was able to tell and to relive emotionally the neglect and frustrations she had experienced in early childhood. She became more and more consciously aware of her own negative and competitive attitude towards her daughter, her husband and her worker.

It should be mentioned that whenever the worker showed Mrs. Y. the operation of destructive impulses in relationship to her child or the therapist, the results were invariably a greater need on the part of Mrs. Y. to deny such direct interpretation of her hostility. These interpretations merely increased the feelings of her own worthlessness. A direct expression of hostility was fraught with direct consequences because it would mean the loss of much needed love from a maternal figure. In this case, the worker took over Mrs. Y's hostility which she dared not recognize in herself and which had to be repudiated.

When the worker, mirroring the patient, presented herself in a destructive, inconsiderate, "worthless" way or even as a failure, the patient was no longer confronted by an omnipotent mother figure who protected her against the dangers of life. Mrs. Y. had to adopt immediately, against the worker's apparently hopeless outlook and helplessness, a constructive attitude and a resourcefulness which overcame her former paralyzing dependence. She now could begin to feel neglected by a mother figure and could also feel her resentment over such neglect, but also--and without feelings of guilt--could develop a resourceful attitude which helped her to change the situation.

Thus, it was not merely the release of hostility or competitive strivings which improved the therapeutic situation. At some stages in her therapy Mrs. Y. had always been able to express hostility, but all these aggressive outbursts would only increase guilt, lead to self-accusation, self-punishment and increased feelings of helplessness. This occurred because the mother was seen only as a powerful figure and not also as a helpless person. When Mrs. Y. mobilized herself, could see and use herself more realistically and became able to change a situation in her life constructively, self-reproaches and severe super-ego pressures were relieved. This in turn, enabled Mrs. Y. to acknowledge destructive urges which then became accessible to therapeutic investigation.

Discussion

The treatment approach applied in the case of Mrs. Y. may invite a number of criticisms. For example, it might be alleged to represent a deliberate attempt on the worker's part ot utilize the patient's negative suggestibility and thus effect no change in the patient's basic problems. Another objection might be that the therapist runs the risk of self-defeat when he echoes the pessimistic attitude a patient may reveal. The patient may counter such a pessimistic therapist by stating: "Maybe you are right and I cannot change, but if so, why should treatment continue?" Sensibilities may be shocked when we hear the worker suggest a divorce or hospitalization in a mental institution. Such an attitude, for a therapist, seems highly unusual. We ordinarily expect therapists to be supportive and we are not easily reconciled to the idea of a therapist who does not hold out the promise of help.

The surprised reaction with which Mrs. Y. responded to the attitude of the worker should occasion no surprise. The patient had not expected to encounter her own mirror image in the behavior and utterances of the worker. Instead of meeting an expected version of her idealized self, Mrs. Y. met a worker who did not promise help, would not play the omnipotent mother, but rather presented herself as helpless and as a failure. An idealized picture of a mother figure was needed by the patient to maintain her own defense of helplessness but a worker who apparently could refuse help had to appear, with a reaction of shock, as destructive in the patient's eyes.

One may point out that the worker's attitude made it possible for the patient to "project" onto the worker her own destructive wishes and, after seeing them externalized, became able to turn against the worker.

Evidently, Mrs. Y. was unconsciously wishing to mistreat her husband when she constantly complained about him. Her unconscious destructive intent toward her daughter became also visible in her fears when she described Linda as "abnormal" and "crazy". Of course, Mrs. Y. was not aware of the destructive wishes behind her complaints. When she stated that her husband never changed or that her daughter would never get better, the worker did not contradict Mrs. Y., did not insist that the family should be kept together, did not hold out hope that her daughter was as normal as any other young girl; but instead said that perhaps the patient was right.

As long as the worker disagreed with the patient and was encouraging, the fiction of a helpful therapist who would deal with all unpalatable aspects of reality could be maintained. If, however, the worker agreed with the patient, the worker became less valuable. Now the patient had to feel and deal with her own aggressive impulses, namely, as to whether she should leave her husband or should send her daughter to a mental institution. The patient, no longer able to cling to a magical solution, had to envision the reality to destruction so vividly portrayed in the attitude of the therapist.

In reviewing this case, it seems that the defense "I am weak, infantile, helpless" was dropped. The purpose of the defense was to protect the patient against her own unconscious destructiveness. Once the patient could feel this destructiveness, after it was dramatically portrayed in the worker, she could no longer give in to her destructiveness. She could feel her destructiveness, but at the same time she was able to react in a constructive fashion.

A consistent attitude of friendliness by the therapist would have deprived the patient of the possibility to dissent. A too-protective approach turns the worker from a therapist into a gratifying parent, with the result that the patient is forced to idealize the worker, do her bidding and suppress and disguise the aggressive reactions to frustration. In the final analysis, the seemingly frustrating attitude of the worker is essentially a therapeutic device designed to help the patient outgrow her resistances against feeling and expressing the aggressive side of her personality. Once the patient can learn to outgrow her defenses against her aggressive impulsivity, treatment may continue along usual lines with the impasse of the 'negative therapeutic reaction' overcome.

At this time, we are not able to say anything more definite or with greater clarification about the resolution of the "negative therapeutic reaction" through special treatment methods. We are aware that we have not been able to elucidate completely the dynamic constellation in our so-called "untreatable" cases. We are also aware how incomplete our efforts have been in exploring the meaning of the treatment approach as applied in the case of Mrs. Y. We believe, however, that the treatment approach we attempted to describe, from a theoretical viewpoint, might be promising in the treatment of certain cases hitherto considered "untreatable."

14. Group Therapy with Parents of Severely Retarded Children: A Preliminary Report

by Arthur Blatt

From Group Psychotherapy, vol. 10, no. 2, June 1957, J. L. Moreno, M.D., Editor; Beacon House, Inc., Publisher. Dr. Blatt originally noted this acknowledgment of the "suggestions and counsel of J. Michaels, M.D., Associate Medical Director of the Shield of David in the preparation of this paper."

Introduction

The Shield of David is a psychiatric clinic and day school essentially geared and devoted to the problems of the severely retarded child who is not acceptable in the Public School system because of low I.Q. Children, ages 4-12, are admitted to the day school upon the completion of a diagnostic-team study and the recommendation of a staff treatment conference. The diagnostic study consists of intake interviews by social service, medical, psychological and speech examinations, observations of the child in group activities and a psychiatric consultation when deemed necessary. All medical, psychological and psychiatric data available from past studies are obtained. A staff conference is then held and the treatment plan for the child and for the parents is proposed.

It became apparent, in the course of our work, that most children could not derive maximum benefit from the school program without simultaneous help for the parents to understand their own feelings and attitudes toward the children. Therefore, a counselling and therapy program was initiated to meet the needs of the parents. In this paper we wish to present a preliminary report on some of the experiences and problems encountered in the treatment of parents in group therapy. A group therapy program was initiated with the psychiatrist and psychologist conducting individual groups. This study is based on experience with twelve such groups over a two-year period.

Method

Group therapy as a therapeutic medium was utilized because of theoretical and practical considerations. It was felt that the commonable experiences with the retarded child would make for an "in-group" situation which would enable the parents to speak freely of their attitudes and feelings about the child. This "in-group" situation would also facilitate verbalization by the more insecure, defended parents who had socially isolated themselves, as well as orient more realistically the assertive, expansive parents who tended to deny the reality and seriousness of their own and the child's status. The defended, insecure parents on hearing expressed feelings and attitudes which they had suppressed because of shame and/or guilt would be aided in more freely expressing themselves.

We endeavored to have couple groups. It was felt that by having husband and wife in the same group, we could possibly establish personal communication, emotional rapport, consistency in the handling of the child and a deeper appreciation of each other's feelings. It was also felt that the placement of the parents in the same group would enable them to utilize the group therapist positively and not as a weapon against each other.

Our primary goal in the group was the realization by the parents that their own emotional status, attitudes and feelings affected the child-parent relationship, thereby affecting the maximal growth of the child.

The number of members in the group and the length of the group sessions was arrived at arbitrarily. The group enrollment initially was not formally fixed and varied from 8-14 members. At the present time it is felt that a maximum enrollment of 10 members constitutes a feasible working group. The group met once a week for not more than 20 weeks. The session lasted an hour and a half. Whenever possible the groups were made up of couples, but it was found that an all-mothers group was unavoidable and inevitable.

The recommendation for participation in group therapy is made at the staff conference by the psychiatric consultant. In many cases group placement is deferred until the social worker clarifies with the parents the purpose and goals of group therapy and an initial resistance to "telling all those people my problems" is worked through. It is apparent that parent interest is a primary criterion for group placement. Initially intellectual levels were disregarded in group placement, but this was found to be disruptive, unproductive and unprofitable for the group. At the present time groups are homogeneous only in intellectual level and the fact of having a retarded child. Race, color, religious belief are disregarded as well as social, financial background. Ambulatory psychotics, psychopaths and severely neurotically disturbed parents are excluded from group therapy.

Discussion

The primary difficulty noted in our group therapy program was the problem of adhering to the therapeutic goal, i.e., an understanding of one's attitudes and feelings toward the retarded child. This was frustrating to parents who wanted to go further into an exploration of themselves aside from the child, and frightening to parents who were threatened by the verbalizing of one's feelings and attitudes about the child. The former view was exemplified in statements such as:

> I feel the questions should be more personal and bring out feelings about each other as well as the child.
>
> If there was some way to get people to really open up, I think we'd all gain a great deal more.
>
> We skirted basic problems but never really touched them.

The latter view was expressed in statements such as:

> I would like more professional advice such as lectures by doctors in various fields.

> I feel I would like outlined discussions.
>
> I would like films of institutional life as well as films of school life for children of lower levels.

This divergence of opinions suggests the need for a more careful screening of parental needs to determine their ability and availability to utilize group therapy meaningfully. These early experiences with group therapy indicate very clearly the need for various group goals based on the ego-strength (capacities), ego defenses and needs of the individual.

Another bar to the therapeutic process was the viewing of the therapist by the parents as an outsider who could not possibly understand their problems. This appeared to be a hostile projection against all professional people because of their past experiences with workers in the field, and a defense against the therapeutic process itself. Statements such as "You can't know unless you have a retarded child," "I know the books say . . ." and "You're here because of your training and background" were usually elicited whenever the parent had been disturbed by the therapist's interpretations or explanations. In a group psychotherapy situation this could be treated as a resistance and dealt with accordingly, but in our therapeutic paradigm, the therapist would have to wait for another member of the group to literally "resay" the interpretation before it was acceptable.

> Mr. R. had read a great deal on the problem of retardation and was quite active in a local organization dealing with retarded children. At the group sessions he utilized his humor and wit to dispel the seriousness of the various feelings expressed by other group members. The therapist at one session pointed out that he seemed to take the group sessions as a joke. He denied this, noting "Psychologists are always reading things into what people say." At a subsequent session a few parents, piqued by his humor, pointed out to him that he was acting like a clown. The following session he noted, "I guess I joke around a great deal because it hurts when I get serious about my child."

It has been our experience that those parents who resort to divinity as a protection against their own feelings are difficult candidates for group therapy. As long as the group does not threaten their defense, they will remain in group and maintain an attitude of aloof, disinterested spectators. When other members question them as to "why they feel that it was God's will," they do not show up for further group meetings and rationalize their absence at meetings. They do not say they do not want to be in group but rather that they just can't seem to "find the time," no adequate baby sitters, "the weather was poor," etc., until such time as they are dropped from group. Their resorting to God may not at all be related to their active participation and belief in the religion and as such represents a personality problem. Often they will misrepresent the precepts of the religion as saying they must keep the child at home. It is our impression that these parents require intensive individual therapy and should not be placed in a group therapy situation.

Our observations indicate that many parents have intense, aggressive impulses toward the child. Although these feelings may be effectively suppressed the individuals are nevertheless left with a feeling of guilt. We have found that quite often the need to release these feelings will come out in a dream which the parent feels impelled to tell the group. This generally releases the group whose perception of the dream is echoed in their own psyche.

> After a few sessions spent on a discussion of the parent's acceptance of the child and in which no mention was made of hostile feelings toward the child, Mrs. L. felt that she had to tell the group a dream she had. "I dreamed I was on the elevated subway platform with L. When the train came in, I waited until the doors were almost closed and jumped in, leaving him on the platform. I waved to him and suddenly felt that I wanted to get out of the train." When one parent noted, "It sounds as if you want to get away from him," this opened up a flood of anger and resentment toward the child. This first expression of anger and resentment enabled other members to express their hostile feelings toward the children.
>
> In another group, Mrs. R. casually mentioned to the group that she had a dream which was annoying

> her. She noted, "I dreamed that R. fell out of the window and was holding on to the window sash. I watched him and then slammed shut the window on his fingers." The meaning of the dream was clear to her, but what impelled her to tell the dream to the group was the need for catharsis with its concomitant reduction of anxiety. The group response was immediate with other members speaking about their own aggressive impulses toward their children.

It seems to be inevitable that the sessions following such a release are essentially tense but quiet with the members seeming to be apprehensive of each other. At this point the explanation by the therapist that parents who have "normal" children will also feel the way they do at time, clears the air for further therapeutic progress. We have also noted that in these parents, there is a quality of "superforgivingness," a tendency to idealize themselves with more than the normal allotment of forgiveness as a reaction formation to guilt over hostile feelings toward the child. This becomes an almost circular mechanism in that the least suggestion of guilt or hostility incurs an increased need to forgive which in turn increases their inner vindictive drives.

One of the major problems that has to be dealt with in group is that of externalization, i.e., the feeling of group members that the environment they are in is hostile toward the child. Most often this is found to be an externalization of the parents' feeling that the people staring at the child are staring at them. This activates their own neurotic structure and inadequacies which they do not have to face since the problem is foisted on to the child.

> Mrs. N. noted in group her feelings of hostility toward a strange woman who kept staring at her daughter while at a public swimming pool. As she talked it became apparent to the group that her feeling was that she was the one who was embarrassed and in effect felt that the woman was looking at her. Even more fundamentally it was she herself who was staring with hostility at the child and externalizing these feelings.

It has been our observation in group that the guilt

over having a retarded child is intimately related to the trauma experienced by the parents to their own self-concept.

In presenting the following case summaries, we will illustrate how the inability of the parents to utilize group therapy positively was a function of their personality structure and to show successful utilization of group therapy by parents.

> Case #1. Mr. and Mrs. R., age 47 and 46 respectively, began Group Therapy February, 1955 in separate groups. A psychiatric consultation noted that "Mr. R. is predominantly of a self-effacing character structure. In a group, Mr. R. may find it possible to be more self-expressive." "Mrs. R. displayed considerable tension characterized by psychomotor activity. She is constantly on the defensive and rationalizes quickly and well. It is conceivable that Mrs. R. in her aggressive, opinionated and self-righteous attitude would act as a stimulus for the group as well as perhaps acquiring further insights for herself."
>
> Their child, aged 11, an only child, is severely mentally retarded, non-verbal and physically handicapped. After 2 years of treatment of the child, the concensus of staff opinion was that the child ought to be placed in a state school. Mr. and Mrs. R. are against placing the child away from home.

The course of group therapy for Mrs. R. who was in a predominantly mothers' group was stormy. Although she would orally argue with the group, in practice she modified some of her rigid practices with the child, e.g., she stopped giving the child suppositories to regulate his bowel movements, and instead of constantly carrying or wheeling him around, gave him more freedom to walk. In spite of some modifications in practice she still felt that she had to defend her position as a harrassed mother who was obligated to help the child.

Mr. R. attended a primarily couples' group. His attendance at group was marked by a stolid silence or monosyllabic responses to questions directed at him by the group. His response to friendly overtures on the part of group members was to deliberately shut them out. The only breakthrough occurred once when the group discussed a film on institutions they had seen on T.V. At this time Mr. R. insisted that he would not place R. and in the next breath resignedly noted that someday it would have to be.

In both parents it became obvious that their rigid character structures would not be able to tolerate an exposure of their inner hostility toward the child. Hardship and difficulty with the child were idealized into virtues and was experienced as a not uncommon "masochistic" mechanism. It is felt that this reversal is usually an indication of extensive hostility toward the child which is suppressed and reversed into a martyr-like acceptance of the child. Since the group threatens the reality of their views they defend themselves (1) by an active offensive toward the group, which diverts the group from themselves, (2) a passive withdrawal from what is going on in the group and (3) a complete refusal to be in group.

> Case #II. Mr. and Mrs. J., age 34 and 33 respectively, began Group Therapy together November, 1955. At the Staff Conference it was noted that "there appeared to be some familial difficulty in that despite the mother's intensive interest, the father is a rather withdrawn and resigned type of individual. This generates further difficulty for the mother and it is felt that both parents can derive considerable help from group."
>
> Their child, aged 5, is the older of two siblings. She is a moderately retarded mongoloid who has shown progress in the 1 1/2 years she has attended schools.

Their course of treatment together in group led to many open arguments and denouncements of not caring for the child. When they first came to group they had still not let their own parents know that the child was retarded. They were able to work out many of their feelings of guilt, shame and frustration over having a retarded child and ceased to blame each other for the child's condition. As they explored their feelings about the child and each other, they found that they could more freely communicate with each other in a way that they never had before. Mr. J. became more emotionally involved with the child and what was happening at home. They were able to inform their parents of the child's condition and felt "as if a load of bricks was taken off my back." These parents were able to utilize the group for the goals that were set for the group. Through catharsis, emotionally facing each other, identification with the feelings of other group members, support from the group members and from the therapist, they were able to derive maximal benefit from the group.

Summary

For the past two years a group therapy program with parents of children who are severely mentally retarded has been held at the Shield of David. We have found this to be a meaningful therapeutic medium for many parents. It is unique in that it allows for an emotional rapport between parents that enables them to discuss their feelings more extensively in a shorter period of time than it would take in individual treatment.

At the present time, we foresee the need for three types of groups:

I. Educational Group Counselling: to include those parents whole defenses are fragile and brittle. This group would have as its core matter the techniques of child rearing and development.

II. Group Counselling: to include those parents whose ego strength is sufficiently strong to explore their attitudes and feelings as related to the child.

III. Group Psychotherapy: to include those parents who indicate a desire to delve into their own emotions and feelings. This would only incidentally be related to the child.

The need for a more formal psychotherapeutic group became apparent as it was found that oftimes the problems of the parents transcended the immediate problems with the child, that many parents used the problem with the child as a protection against seeing their own psychic problems and/ or as a protection against the possible dissolution of a poor marital situation.

The group structure can be used meaningfully for most parents if the group goals are structured to meet the needs and capacities of the parents.

15. Some Considerations on the Therapeutic Neglect of Fathers in Child Guidance

by Henry U. Grunebaum and Herbert S. Strean

From *Journal of Child Psychology and Psychiatry,* vol. 5, 1964. Reprinted with the permission of Pergamon Press.

Introduction

Almost sixty years ago a small boy suffering from an animal phobia began psychoanalytic psychotherapy. He was later referred to as Little Hans. For our present purposes it is of particular interest that he was treated by his father under the supervision of Sigmund Freud.

Today, despite the fact that the child guidance movement has come of age, the father is still infrequently part of his child's therapeutic program. We are impressed with a nearly universal phenomenon, namely, that almost all clinics find it difficult to involve fathers in treatment. Many fathers resist treatment and/or guidance, and when they finally agree to participate in a therapeutic plan their attrition rate is higher than that of either mothers or children. A review of the literature demonstrates that throughout the history of the child guidance movement pleas have been made that fathers be considered seriously as treatment candidates; these pleas have been all too frequently unheeded.

We aim to discuss the difficulties involved in treating fathers, within the framework of the history and theoretical orientation of the child guidance movement. To be considered also is the psychology of fathers of disturbed children and the problems in their therapy. Case examples will be used to illustrate typical impasses in the relationship between clinic, father and therapist. Our work is based on our experiences in treating fathers individually and in groups, at two geographically separated clinics for the treatment of pre-school children.

The Child Guidance Movement and the Father

Richmond (1917) wrote that in planning treatment there is need to consider "the Family Group. . . which includes all who share a common table." Yet Towle (1930) wrote that

> . . . "It is generally agreed that fathers have been left too much out of the picture. This has occurred largely through the inconvenience in reaching them and the scarcity of their time (not to mention our time). . . . The fine point of seeing the father first, and making him the focus of treatment if the case indicates this need, is not a general practice. This may be due to the inconvenience, in spite of the realization of his significance in the situation.

Other articles echoing the need for including fathers in a diagnostic evaluation recur throughout the forties. Pollak (1956), in a review, noted that the attitude towards the father had not changed in thirty years and that it was still a general feature of child guidance clinics for fathers not to be seen. He stated, "The mother is practically the only factor besides the child's personality structure to which attention is paid in treatment if not in diagnosis."

Burgum (1942), in a pioneer article, was the first to document a common observation: a change in family dynamics may benefit one member but have adverse effects on another. She commented further

> Occasional murmurs about the father as a factor in child guidance treatment echo through the field. The fact that the mother is the person most involved in responsibility for the child and his difficulties, and also most accessible in terms of her own time and agency working hours, tends to focus attention on her both in diagnostic and treatment considerations. The father is not entirely neglected, yet the full significance of

> his role in the treatment situation is rarely adequately realized. . . .

During the forties and fifties fathers were almost exclusively seen through their wives' eyes. There are, however, a few exceptions noted in the literature. Beron (1944) noted that fathers who applied for treatment for their children were usually passive men, struggling against their passivity. The fact that they applied for treatment for their children often threatened the mother of the child and made her treatment more difficult. Sternberg (1951) found that the parent who initiated the treatment had the healthier relationship with the child, stayed in treatment longer, made greater therapeutic gains, projected less on to the child, and focused more directly in the therapy on his relationship with the child.[1]

Some of the difficulties in treating fathers were noted by Staver (1944). She concluded that the clinic activates a wish to confess weakness in men who may be defending against it, and that "it may also be that these fathers would find a man less threatening than a woman case worker." Walton (1940) found that the father used the clinic to express his own feelings of "inferiority or insecurity" and that the treatment of the child lasted longer in those cases in which the father came to treatment frequently. She also found that there was a higher proportion of success in those cases in which the fathers participated.

Most recently, Bell, Trieschman and Vogel (1961) discuss at length the bias towards a consideration of only the mother-child relationship in etiological formulations, and the resistances to treatment of the working-class father who expects to give formal assent to the treatment of his child but that he, himself, will not be directly involved in the therapeutic plan. This father also expects to be judged, found wanting, told what to do, and sent on his way. The authors discuss the sources of resistance of these fathers in terms of the general role dispositions of working-class people, contrasting these with those of the more middle-class therapist.

There is a tendency for working-class fathers of disturbed children to show a more rigid division of labor between men and women than is usual. Bell _et al._ (1961) feel that this penomenon relates to maintenance of masculine identity by these particular fathers in order to avoid contact with feminine preoccupations. Treatment is seen by them as a feminine concern and is therefore especially threatening. The importance of the coalition of mother and child against the father is also discussed. They further note, as did Staver (1944), that "The clinic is a place where there are many women and few men."

While Bell et al. consider only working-class fathers, it has been our experience that these features are frequently present in middle-class and upper-class fathers, with whom we are more familiar. In fact, aside from a certain ability to intellectualize on the part of the middle-class father and a propensity for action on the part of the lower-class father, it appears that many of the problems encountered in the treatment of fathers are similar, regardless of class.

Who Will Treat the Father and How

The child guidance movement began with the child as patient, and only later did the need for the participation of the mother evolve. First the mother was an informant, and later she was seen as a person with problems in her own right. The mother was the logical parent[2] to be seen because she brought the child to the clinic and, therefore, was available. She spent the most time with the child and could thus give the kind of information which would aid the child's therapist. Furthermore, she could be given advice to follow at home which might help the child. Gradually it became apparent that the mother herself needed treatment and needed it for reasons which were related to the child's problem, and thus casework with mothers evolved.

While perhaps Freud himself focused more on fathers than on mothers it may be asked if certain aspects of the influence of psychoanalysis, as it became an important theoretical and therapeutic framework for the child guidance clinic, did not discourage the treatment of fathers. Psychoanalytic treatment is most clearly developed for adult outpatient neurotics, and its transfer to the child guidance clinic has led to certain difficulties. The treatment focus is on intrapsychic conflict, rather than on family relationships, and the method is a highly individual one. This treatment method offers much to the independent adult who can to a considerable extent choose and influence his environment, but it may well run into difficulty with the more dependent child, whose environment tends to influence and control him considerably.

Psychoanalytic theory is one of intrapsychic dynamics rather than of group interactions and is not pre-eminently a field theory. It tends to concentrate on dyads, or relationships between two people, and since it is evident that the earliest and most significant relationship of the child is with his mother, psychoanalytic theory provides a better rationale for including the mother than the father. It is evident, however, that if one takes a point of view which looks at the family as a field of forces (Spiegel and Bell, 1957; Meissner, 1964) one is impressed with how a mother's influence on the child will be intimately related to her relationship with her husband, and that she may not be able to deal with her child differently unless the family changes in its entirety. The influence of psychoanalytic treatment and theory is difficult to discuss, particularly in view of the many minority influences within it. However, it may be said that, in the main, it has emphasized the treatment of the individual child patient by the individual therapist, and the strength of the child's attachment to his mother, and has not specifically encouraged the treatment of fathers.[3]

Pollak (1956), whose work we have referred to frequently, comments at length on the problems encountered in the application of psychoanalytic theory to the family and to the problems of disturbed children. He feels there is great need for a field theory and attempts in part to adapt certain views of Lewin (1933). Whether or not the utilization of field theory is necessary, it is obvious that throughout the history of the child guidance movement pleas have been made that fathers be seen in diagnosis and offered treatment. Yet the clinic team of social worker and child psychiatrist evolved without a specific person to treat the father, nor has the predominant theoretical orientation provided a clearcut rationale for treating him. The current child guidance approach is oriented towards individual conflict seen in terms of dyads rather than as occurring within the patient's psychological field, including all the significant emotional forces within it.

Why Treat the Father?

A finding that most child guidance clinics report is that almost 70 per cent of their treatment cases are boys (U.S. Department of Health, Education and Welfare, 1962). Closer scrutiny reveals that many of these male youngsters suffer from ego problems where lacunae in masculine identification exist. The father is often experienced as withdrawn and passive by his family, and frequently there is a coalition between child and mother from which he is excluded. In healthy families the opposite has been noted by Hoffman (1961), who states, "When the father is more powerful than the mother, disciplines his children, and has a warm companionship with them, the boys, and to a lesser extent, the girls, will have self-confidence, feel accepted by others, show positive assertiveness in their peer group, have skills, like others, be liked, and exert influence upon others."

Most of the fathers seen for diagnosis and treatment at child guidance clinics appear as rather passive, withdrawn men who interact little with their sons. Is it any wonder, then, that they deny their passivity and need for help, and avoid the clinic which they see as a predominantly feminine atmosphere, as Staver (1944), Bell *et al.* (1961), and Seeley *et al.* (1956).[4] have noted? In addition, it is frequently the case that their wives seek and use their sons as substitutes for their passive husbands. The mother excludes the father because of her desire to perpetuate a coalition with her child or children in which she has, and from which she derives, a certain degree of power. She also feels that she cannot get what she needs from her passive husband, yet would be thwarted were he to assert himself.[5] However, is it not then vital for the father to be involved in treatment, since if he is withdrawn and passive his exclusion from it must merely perpetuate familial neurotic patterns?

A clinical example may clarify these issues:

> Sally B. was brought to the clinic by her mother, but without very much consultation with her father. Feeling excluded by his wife and daughter, Mr. B. arrived for his first clinical consultation angry, belligerent, and said, "I don't need to consult anybody

about myself and my family; I can do it by myself." He was clearly making the therapist the passive recipient of what he had experienced with his wife and daughter. In this situation, the interviewer was sensitive and responsive to Mr. B.'s underlying need. He remarked, "Mr. B., you certainly are a very self-sufficient man. It is regrettable that you won't have anything to do with me because I need you to help your daughter and wife." Looking surprised and a little shocked, Mr. B. asked provocatively, "What in the dickens do you need me for?" To this the therapist responded, "To treat a child every therapist needs a father to guide him." The therapist was able to speak securely about his own dependent feelings which Mr. B. feared in himself. Also, he gratified the wish that Mr. B.'s wife had frustrated--the wish to be needed. Feeling needed, Mr. B. could discuss with his therapist his feeling of desertion by his wife and daughter. With support and encouragement he could begin to explore his own role in provoking and inducing some of his wife's behavior towards him. Sally's conflicts, it should be noted, were in many ways a reactive response to the marital instability which both parents could now face.

The Father and His Therapist

We may now look at the problems from the point of view of the therapist. The resistances against treatment used by the fathers manifest themselves in their remarks about their lack of knowledge of the child, the inconvenience of coming to appointments at hours which conflict with work, and their lack of influence upon the child.

Psychotherapists are, however, used to overcoming resistances. While the history of the child guidance movement and the evolution of the team has led to certain practical difficulties in finding a therapist for a father, perhaps these obstacles are not insurmountable. Perhaps some of the resistances come from within ourselves. We may wonder if some of the feelings of the clinic in treating parents in general, and fathers in particular, do not result from a natural desire to help the sick child in emotional distress who is seen as the sad and inevitable product of a hostile and ungratifying environment. The therapist may thus wish to "make it up" to the unfortunate child.

Ekstein (1962) has recently written

> Child psychiatrists usually have a kind of identification with their patients which makes the therapists natural enemies of the child's parents. He is out to prove that he can do better than the child's parents, that he must undo the wrong inflicted on the child. He sees many of his difficulties in treating children as difficulties of the parents who interfere with and sabotage the treatment.

Parents must be involed in the treatment plan, then, in order to prevent this kind of sabotage.

Since the child guidance clinic is largely staffed by women it may be that this leads to greater conflict in working with clients of the opposite sex. Pollak (1956) comments

> It might prove fruitful to give some attention to the possibility that women social workers, women clinicians, and women psychiatrists may prefer to associate with women clients or women patients because they recognize them as of like kind with themselves, and thus the worker determines the 'parent' with whom she prefers to associate in the clinical contacts.

While it may be true, as Pollak suggests, that therapists prefer to work with clients of the same sex, it would seem just as likely that they might prefer clients of the other sex. Certainly there are few, if any, clearcut indications for determining by age, sex, or diagnosis whether a patient will do better with a male or female therapist. All experienced workers have had both successes and failures with patients of each sex. We would suggest, however, that fathers are not patients, at least when first seen at a clinic. They come for help, not with the internalized problems causing them anxiety, guilt, or depression, but rather because of their children's problems. As such they come because of difficulties in being fathers. If they can be helped to perform better in their roles as fathers, a therapeutic alliance can often be built which will gradually permit them to see themselves as patients with neurotic problems in their own right. This process, however, depends heavily on their being assisted to be better fathers. Helping a father may well be easier for a therapist who is familiar with the role rather than one who is not. We would therefore hypothesize that it is not that the child guidance worker chooses the sex of the patient she works with, but rather that she is influenced, among other things, by the natural desire to help those whom she feels best able to help.

Child therapists may wish to be both parents to a child. They are likely to be more threatened by the person who is the natural leader of the family, namely the father, than by the mother. The mother may be seen by a social worker, and thus the child psychiatrist has both the child to help and the family to lead.

This viewpoint is supported by Ekstein (1962) who notes, "The therapist's basic attitudes towards parents, frequently towards all adults (including his supervisor), are rebellious ones." If the therapist is a rebellious person, one of the people he may need to rebel against is the natural leader of the family who has abrogated his function, namely the father. For instance, Rubenstein and Levitt (1957) found that the therapist may often ally himself with the unconscious-aggressive striving of adolescent boys, particularly as these lead to acting-out defiance of the father. If may, therefore, make sense that the child's therapist will have feelings that the child has been led astray and that he, the therapist alone, without the father's participation, will lead him aright psychotherapeutically.

On the other hand, if the emphasis in treatment is upon support and therapeutic work within the existing leadership of the family the father must be seen in treatment. However, because of his own passivity and need to abdicate the leadership, there is a lacuna into which the child guidance worker can easily fall. The mother brings the child for treatment, and she then appears as the leader of the family to all concerned.

An occurrence repeatedly noted is that in the father's

absence from the clinic the therapist becomes the father surrogate, or family leader, alienating the father and disrupting the family equilibrium further. An example will illustrate this pitfall:

> Jerry C., aged eleven, was referred to a child guidance clinic by school personnel because he appeared "sissified, effeminate, passive and old-maidish." Clinical findings revealed a strong symbiotic relationship between mother and child, with both engaged in a highly seductive relationship. Jerry and his mother slept together frequently, particularly in the father's absence. The father saw "nothing wrong with the boy," but the mother felt "that the school must know something and I don't want to raise him to be a homosexual." Because of the strong symbiotic relationship between mother and son it was felt that both parties should be seen by the same therapist because a too-rapid separation initially might be intolerable. No treatment was offered the father. In treatment both the mother and son formed relationships to the therapist similar to their relationship to one another: dependent, clinging, unaggressive and unassertive. Their aggression went underground as they both enjoyed "a love and be loved relationship" with the therapist. Their interviews brought them both much libidinal satisfaction, but as their treatment went on the father became more withdrawn, came home less frequently, and the marital relationship seriously deteriorated. It was not until the father threatened divorce action that Mrs. C. could begin to explore her role in either the marital or parental relationship. With her treatment less "satisfying" she could begin to direct some of her verbal aggression towards her therapist and begin to "look at my husband."
> With her encouragement Mr. C. was offered and accepted treatment at the clinic.

It is not surprising that the father's image of his position in the family is often shared by those who treat him. We have observed and participated in several situations where the therapists who were working with fathers relegated to themselves, or were relegated, a subordinate position in the therapeutic team. Frequently fathers are treated after clinic hours, partly as a convenience, often with no monetary remuneration, and this treatment is regarded as a "learning experience" rather than as part of the "work week."

One of the writers was asked to supervise the treatment of a father's therapy group which met at the clinic of a wealthy suburban community. Despite the fact that all the members of the group enjoyed substantial incomes, they were not required to pay for the therapeutic experience. When the supervisor investigated this the therapist's response was, "How can I charge them anything when they are coming at night?" When the therapist was told that the men were being provided an experience that was quite convenient for them, therefore perhaps they should pay more than the usual rate, the therapist responded, "Well, I'm not getting paid for this. It's all an experiment."

In this situation the therapist was doing himself an injustice. In effect, he was saying that his therapeutic time and effort were worth very little, perhaps nothing. When he was asked why he accepted a salary for his work with mothers and children he stated that this was "something else." In essence, he was reflecting the self-images of the fathers he was treating, abdicating his own role as a potentially strong figure with whom his patients could identify.

Group Therapy and the Father

Not by chance, the treatment offered fathers is often group psychotherapy. Since it is widely believed that they will not come for treatment during clinic hours, group psychotherapy offers a way of seeing many fathers at once, and using little therapy time after hours. In addition, group psychotherapy is often regarded as "second rate" treatment which may be appropriately offered to "second class" patients. We do not, however, agree that it is a "second rate treatment," and our experiences suggest that it may have certain specific advantages for the fathers we have described as typically seen in child guidance clinics for preschool children (Grunebaum, 1962; Strean, 1962). Not only does the group offer what the father needs, but his needs and the characteristics of group psychotherapists seem to coincide.

We are impressed that group psychotherapists differ somewhat from other therapists. First of all, and most obviously, they have needs to lead--perhaps not so much to rescue--but more to dominate. Secondly, they have needs to work not just with one person but with many. Finally, they appear to have wishes to be active and visible, as group therapy demands. These needs may perhaps explain why many group psychotherapists are also interested in activity therapy, the treatment of psychotics and delinquents. In all these kinds of treatment leadership, activity and visibility are necessary.

The desire to lead a group, to be active and visible, may explain why group psychotherapists are interested in the treatment of fathers. This is appropriate, since leadership, activity, and visibility are precisely what the passive fathers of many disturbed children lack. The group leader is a more appropriate object for identification than the weak, absent, or punitive fathers these men themselves have had in the past.

At times a father's wish not to be seen must be respected. Occasionally, it is necessary to see him less or more frequently than is traditional. We have found fathers' groups, where discussion is more diffused and self-exposure less obligatory, helpful to many resistive fathers, and groups may, in fact, have certain definite advantages for them. It permits men who are often rather passive and isolated to have the experience of belonging to a men's group. Such groups are a natural part of the adolescent's growth into manhood, as for instance scouts, boys' clubs and neighborhood groups. The therapy group thus offers a new opportunity to experience and explore the pitfalls of being a man. It is, however, apparent that the treatment of fathers requires sensitive understanding of their psychology.

Summary

In summary, it appears that throughout the history of the child guidance movement largely unheeded pleas for the treatment of fathers have been made. A review of the literature suggests that the passivity of the fathers, the strength of the mother-child coalition, and the threats posed by the clinic are important factors in making difficult the treatment of fathers. It has been noted that the clinic team does not provide a member specifically delegated to treat fathers, and that its treatment philosophy does not offer clearcut reasons for such therapy. In addition, we have offered certain speculations which may explain the child guidance worker's reluctance to treat the father, in contrast to the interest in him of a group psychotherapist. Reasons are also given why group therapy may be a treatment choice for the father.

In conclusion, we may, in a now familiar plea, ask for a broader perspective in the diagnosis of families. Often we do not know who the child's crucial objects are. We assume too readily that there are his parents, when in cases we have seen they are his grandmother, the housekeeper, and, in one instance, the mother's own nurse, who was now caring for her child. We know far too little of the means by which families cope with, and fail, in their efforts to deal with life tasks. In our present state of knowledge, flexibility of diagnostic approach and treatment is vital. Our theoretical and personal biases must constantly be carefully reviewed.

Notes

1. It is of interest that one of the clinics with which we are associated began in 1963 to encourage both parents to come to the intake interview.

2. In passing we may note that Pollak (1956, p. 202-204) mentions the fascinating use of the singular work "parent" in the literature when "parents" is meant. For instance, Zilboorg (1931) states, "It has become a truism to say that you must frequently treat the parent if you want to help the child who has psychological difficulties." Similar quotes from F. Allen, W. Langford and L. Lowrey are given.

3. In this context we may note that *The Psychoanalytic Study of the Child*, in its volumes to date, has published 17 articles which refer to the "mother" in the title, 6 which refer to "maternal" in the title, and only 1 which refers to the "father" or "paternal" in the title. The latter is an article on a fatherless child.

4. These authors found in a community survey that middle-class fathers see the child guidance clinic and psychotherapy as being part of the woman's world. They state, "For man, effect and achievement are the paramount divisions of classification; for the woman, motive, intent and feeling. . . . It is perhaps more on this ground than on any other that the experts and also some religious leaders (the experts referred to are experts in child guidance and child education) are felt by the men as 'feminine'. The experts, like the women, stress the primacy of inner meanings over outer similarities" (p. 384).

5. We have often heard complaints from the therapists of mothers that they are concerned since the mother is becoming disturbed by her husband's increasing assertiveness as he makes progress in treatment.

References

Bell, Norman W., Trieschman, Albert and Vogel, Ezra (1961) A sociocultural analysis of the resistances of working-class fathers treated in a child psychiatric clinic. Amer. J. Orthopsychiat. 31, 388-405.

Beron, Lillian (1944) Fathers as clients of a child guidance clinic. Smith College Stud. Soc. Work 14. 351-366.

Burgum, Mildred (1942) The father gets worse: A child guidance problem. Amer. J. Orthopsychiat. 12, 474-486.

Ekstein, Rudolf (1962) Special training problems in psychotherapeutic work with psychotic and borderline children. Amer. J. Orthopsychiat. 32, 569-584.

Grunebaum, Henry (1962) Group psychotherapy of fathers: Problems of technique. Brit. J. Med. Psychol. 35, 147-154.

Hoffman, Lois Wladis (1961) The father's role in the family and the child's peer-group adjustment. Merrill Palmer Quart. 7, 97-105.

Lewin, Kurt (1933) Environmental Forces. A Handbook of Child Psychology, Ed. Carl Murchison, Clark University Press, Worcester, Mass., p. 594-595.

Meissner, W. W. (1964) Thinking about the family: Psychiatric aspects. Family Process 3, 1-40.

Pollak, Otto (1956) Integrating Sociological and Psychoanalytic Concepts, An Exploration in Child Psychotherapy. Russell Sage Foundation, New York.

Richards, Mary E. (1948-49) When to include the fathers in child guidance. Smith College Stud. Soc. Work 19, 79-95.

Richmond, Mary (1917) Social Diagnosis. Russell Sage Foundation, New York.

Rubenstein, Benjamin O. and Levitt, Morton (1957) Some observations regarding the role of fathers in child psychotherapy. Bull. Menn. Clinic 21, 16-27.

Seeley, John R., Sim, R. Alexander and Loosley, Elizabeth W. (1956) Crestwood Heights. Basic Books, New York.

Spiegel, John P. and Bell, Norman W. (1957) The family of the psychiatric patient. Am. Handbook of Psychiatry. Ed. Silvano Arieti, p. 114-149. Basic Books, New York.

Staver, Nancy (1944) The use of a child guidance clinic by mother-dominant families. Smith College Stud. Soc. Work 14, 367-388.

Sternberg, Harriet (1951) Fathers who apply for child guidance. Smith College Stud. Soc. Work 22, 53-68.

Strean, Herbert (1962) A means of involving fathers in family treatment--Guidance groups for fathers. Amer. J. Orthopsychiat. 32, 714-727.

Towle, Charlotte (1930) The social worker, in Symposium: The treatment of behavior and personality problems in children. Amer. J. Orthopsychiat. 1, 26-27.

Towle, Charlotte (1941) Social Case Records from Psychiatric Clinics, with Discussion Notes. University of Chicago Press, Chicago, p. 284-312.

U. S. Department of Health, Education and Welfare (1962) Data on Patients of Outpatient Psychiatric Clinics in the United States. U. S. Dept. of Health, Education, and Welfare, Public Health Services, Washington, D. C.

Walton, Elizabeth (1940) The role of the father in treatment at a child guidance clinic. Smith College Stud. Soc. Work 11, 155.

Zilboorg, Gregory (1931) Sidelights in parent-child antagonism. Amer. J. Orthopsychiat. 2, 35-43.

16. Psychotherapy with Children of Psychotherapists

by Herbert S. Strean

From The Psychoanalytic Review, vol. 56, no. 4, Winter 1969. Reprinted by permission.

An occurrence transpiring almost daily in the offices of family agencies, mental hygiene clinics, child guidance centers, and private practitioners is the phenomenon of psychotherapists who enact the roles of patients and clients. Despite the fact that, since the inception of the practice of psychotherapy, the notion that "therapists are people, too" has been held to be virtually axiomatic, there is paucity of published data on what occurs when the psychotherapist and/or members of his family are recipients of professional therapeutic services. The issue of "confidentiality" may certainly be a factor in our lack of literature on the subject; however, we have been trained to edit documents so that the patient's privacy can be insured. The lack of explication and dearth of literature on the participation of professionals in treatment exists within several disciplines, such as in psychoanalysis, psychology, and psychiatry, and even the "didactic" or "training analysis" has received little written systematic exploration despite its ubiquity in psychoanalytic training institutes.[1]

It is reasonable to infer that when cases are reported on specified groups, our diagnostic acumen can often be enhanced and our therapeutic armamentarium enriched. With the recent buttressing of our professional knowledge by the social and behavioral sciences, we have become more sensitive to the dominant values of certain subcultures and ethnic groups. Consequently, when therapeutic intervention occurs, the folkways and mores which affect such areas as child rearing and marital relationships have become part of the treatment plan.[3, 5] Perhaps certain aspects of the "therapeutic subculture" may be clarified by examining some of the results of therapy with therapists. This paper is an attempt to initiate dialogue and eventual research into this neglected and shrouded subject.

During the past decade this writer has been afforded the challenging and interesting opportunity of working with over a dozen youngsters who were offspring of therapists. Because the data which emerged during the study and diagnostic phases were sufficiently similar from case to case and inasmuch as the children's responses to treatment held many features in common, it was felt that certain tentative conclusions could evolve concerning patterns of parent-child relationships among therapists. Our findings could have implications for psychotherapists at large and perhaps for the treatment of similar occupational groups. While the N in our report is small (twelve cases) and the treatment itself all took place at social agencies (child guidance clinics) and private practice in one city, New York, we, nonetheless, are of the opinion that our impressions could serve as a starting point from which others may compare and contrast their own experiences.

The Study Phase

The twelve cases under review represent children of therapists who were analysts, psychologists and social workers with no one subgroup having a disproportional representation. The seven boys and five girls ranged in age from 8 years old to 19 with the mean age being 14. The approach by the parents to the initial intake consultations was almost identical in all cases. The spouse who was the therapist made the first contact over phone, requesting "a special favor" or "a very personal request" which "could not be discussed over the phone." Frequently, the parent considered an office discussion as undesirable and preferred a luncheon meeting or social visit. In most cases, the parent only knew the therapist superficially but over the phone he was told that he, the therapist, "knew something about children" and that was why he was being consulted. When the therapist's office (agency office or private office) was suggested as the locus for discussion of the "personal request," most parents balked and either wished to continue the discussion further over the phone or stated that the professional office was "inappropriate." When their preference for the place of the discussion was even superficially explored, in a couple of cases the therapist was told "to forget it" or "never mind, then."

Consequently, as these parents became better known to the therapist, it was considered appropriate to see them at the place they wished to be seen, at their office, their home, or at a restaurant.

After a few pleasantries about the weather and the hectic pace of their own professional lives, most of the parents would initiate the discussion as follows: "I have something embarrassing to discuss with you but I know you'll understand because you have children of your own! You see, my son (daughter) needs treatment." The parents then went on, in most cases, to give a jargon or "technical" description of their youngsters--"he has a lot of repressed hostility and a powerful superego"; "his Oedipal problem has never been resolved and his phobias certainly tell us that"; "his peer relations are impoverished but his object relations towards adults seem less narcissistic." The parent's own relationship to his child was frequently omitted from the report, and when this was explored the parent would characteristically point out that the child under discussion related very well to him (or her) but "had some difficulty" with the spouse.

In almost all of the cases under consideration, the parents had received some form of treatment themselves (usually from a psychiatrist or a psychoanalyst) and in a few cases were in therapy at the time of their application for help with their child. They "saw no need" in becoming involved in the treatment process inasmuch as the child's "difficulty was internalized." They would welcome occasional "discussions" or "chats."

As the study phase was extended, most parents and children reported that the following cluster of presenting problems were emerging: the youngster, although usually having had a superior record of academic achievement, was now functioning below his potential in school. His usually cheerful façade appeared to be undergoing modification and he was becoming depressed; in two cases there were some suicidal gestures. The youngster's demeanor was described as "irritable," "petulant," "supercilious" and "sarcastic." In most situations he was becoming unapproachable and in virtually every case, "he refused to verbalize his feelings" and was "withdrawing from contact more and more." Frequently, the youngsters were experiencing somatic difficulties (stomach aches, headaches, backaches) which the parent labelled as "emotional" or "psychological."

The parents recoiled from any personal involvement when they were asked to present a developmental history. However, despite the paucity of material offered, certain themes were developed in almost all of the histories. The children were planned and wanted. Most pregnancies were uneventful and the infant emerged as "loveable," "alert" and very "bright." Parents often stated that they had experienced "deprived" childhoods themselves and tended to be "overprotective." Overprotection indeed manifested itself by meeting most of the child's demands, rarely limiting him, and with little overt aggression displayed by either parent or child. Sibling rivalry was common but rarely "intense"; "separations" from the parents were difficult in several cases but almost invariably, "worked through."

During the study phase the child usually was reported as being "very resistant" to coming for his intake interview but the parent "could help him come" and almost always did. The youngster always related very politely in his first interviews, pointed out that he was doing poorly in school but often he "didn't care." When prodded, the child confessed that he was moody and depressed but he usually felt that he "could get over it by himself and didn't need help." However, when the therapist asked if "we should forget about the idea of help," the prospective patient invariably stated, "my parents say I must go." On being told in several cases that maybe the therapist could convince the parents that the applicant shouldn't come for help if he didn't want to, the child often became visibly anxious and brought out "real problems that I need help with" or else extolled the therapist for being "understanding and easy to talk with." In no cases did the youngster drop out in the study phase.

Diagnostic Phase

The material in the study phase usually induced a

diagnostic impression of the parents being genuinely concerned about their children's welfare but not wanting to involve themselves in the treatment plan. Their difficulty in assuming the role set of client[3] was obvious in most cases and in virtually every situation they did not want their own feelings explored. Guilty, embarrassed, and anxious about their own contributions to their child's emotional difficulties, they defended themselves by intellectualization, denial, and by professionalizing their own contacts with the therapist. Conflicted because the therapist might eventually function in loco parentis, the majority of parents under examination were impelled to exhibit their own diagnostic prowess and frequently suggested treatment plans for their children to the therapist.[4]

Diagnostically, it appeared that the parents' anxiety and feeling of vulnerability as parents emerged in their need to control the therapy by not having their own pathology exposed. Their insistence upon having the initial consultation regarding their children almost any place other than the therapist's office was recognized as a strong resistance to assuming the patient role vis-à-vis the therapist. It appeared that whatever intrapsychic conflicts they had, the parents did not want them to emerge in their contact with the child's therapist. This attempt to abdicate some psychological responsibility as a parent also appeared in the parents' major defensive maneuver in their relationships with their children--these parents were overly intellectualized in their contacts with their children and tended to control them by "psychoanalytic interpretation." In many ways, then, the parents did not feel free to interact spontaneously with their children and treated them like therapeutic subjects.

The parents' resistance to involvement as clients was mirrored by their children who also "could get along by themselves." Although asking for help, parents and children "did not need it," thus demonstrating much ambivalence regarding the expression of dependency and conflict about the need for professional assistance. The most obvious feature of the parents under examination was their oversolicitude toward their youngsters, rather extreme indulgence, and the consequent squelching of the child's assertiveness and agression. It became clear that the child, who was often described as a "friend" or "pal," was so dependent upon his parents that to oppose or disagree with them would result in overpowering guilt. As a youngster moved toward more autonomy and individuality, he experienced his separations as attacks on his parents and therefore had to retreat with guilt and depression. Although he did not want to see the therapist, who inevitably reminded him of his parents from whom he wished to separate and towards whom he wished to aggress, he felt compelled to obey his parents' command to receive help. As with school, towards which the child had much contempt, he attended treatment interviews compulsively and obediently.

The children most often could be clinically diagnosed as either obsessive character disorders or obsessive compulsive neurotics. While having many ego resources, superego pressures and strong id wishes threw them into much conflict as they attempted to assert themselves. Their depressed affect could be interpreted as aggression turned inward and their academic failures could be seen as unconscious aggressive acts which yielded punishment. Hence, their sadomasochistic orientation was intense as was their pervasive ambivalence.

It will be gleaned from the study data that the dearth of material on the parents, particularly material on the story of their own lives and specifically, data on their marriage, prevented the therapist from even attempting to make a comprehensive family diagnosis. Material on relationships to the extended family and on other significant interpersonal relationships was also sparse.

The Treatment Phase

In virtually every case situation the child was seen on a once- or twice-weekly basis, most frequently coming to his interviews accompanied by no one. Efforts to work with the parents at significant times were usually rejected politely by the latter but they all continued to "support the idea of the child's treatment," seeing that he attended his interviews and always making sure that fees were paid.

The children initially came to all of their sessions on time and related to the therapist in a polite but distant manner. They frequently discussed their interests in television, books and sports and the therapist inevitably joined them in these discussions by asking questions and sharing their enthusiasms. These superficial tête-à-têtes lasted only a few weeks and were always followed by complaints about teachers and parents. The hostile remarks towards teachers usually involved themes of excessive demands by the latter, lack of interest by the teachers and too much distance. When these complaints were received neutrally, the children then launched long expressions of anger and vitriolic displays towards their parents.

Parents were frequently labelled "unfair." They didn't provide for a second television set, a second phone, sufficient clothes, or for the child's own car. The parents did not allow the youngster to "stay up past midnight," "did not give more than $3 a week for an allowance" and "were too interested in my school work and friends." During this period of bellowing about parents and school, the parents frequently called the therapist to report that the youngster was appearing less depressed, functioning better in school and appearing less petulant.

Inevitably, the children would want to test the therapist's stance as to whether he "was taking sides," and the fear was that the therapist would be for the parents or against them. This took the form of: "Do you think I'm right about wanting more allowance?"; "Don't you agree that I should have my own car?" or "Why can't you tell my mother that she should be satisfied with my getting C's in school?" When questions were not answered but were either reflected or interpreted, the youngsters experienced this as a frustration and commenced to aggress towards the therapist. "I don't want you to take sides, you're wrong about that, just answer me!" was a typical exhortation. Often the therapist asked, "Why should I give you what you want when you want it?" or, "Why do I have to answer your question?" and the youngster became furious at the therapist for not immediately gratifying him. A period of constant badgering of the therapist with contemptuous remarks always followed for several months, with a concommitant avoidance of conflicts or complaints about parents and teachers.

The youngsters, contrary to the therapist's expectations, did not react with guilt or depression after or during their aggressive displays towards him. Rather, they continued to improve in school, related with more maturity towards their parents and essentially improved their over-all adaptation. When they were asked how come it didn't get them upset to get angry at the therapist, although they often felt guilty toward their parents after hostile outbursts, many of the children responded with sentiments similar to the following: "You see, you are not a goody-goody. As a matter of fact, you don't appear kind of nice, so I don't have to worry about treating you nicely!" One youngster reflected, "You only get upset or guilty when you think the adult can't take it or gets hurt. You don't seem to want me to love you."

Many of the children after a year or a year-and-a-half of treatment wished to quit treatment. They *never* said that the therapist had helped them or that they were functioning better, but instead the wish almost always took an aggressive and hostile form: "I don't particularly want to talk to *you* every week; I've got better things to do"; "While I must admit that I enjoy ranking you out, it is beginning to get boring"; "You know, you don't give me anything!" At this phase of treatment they didn't "care what my father or mother thinks about my seeing you, I'm quitting!" Frequently, they contended "that paying this agency (or the therapist) money, is a waste." One youngster went so far as to say, "I would rather see my parents buy a book for *themselves* or go to the theater than pay you!"

While the youngsters were attempting to separate from the therapist, they occasionally brought in expressions of endorsement from their parents who most frequently stated, "It's up to you and Strean to work it out!" The child usually set the date of termination and kept his own word.

Follow-Up Phase

In ten of the twelve cases under discussion, the parents stayed in telephone or social communication with the therapist after termination. While the therapist was initially and for some time suspicious of reports of their children's sustained and improved functioning, particularly because so many of the youngsters left in anger, some understanding of the process slowly evolved. The youngsters rarely mentioned their treatment experience to their parents and when they did, the therapist was usually described as "a jerk," "a namby-pamby," a "ninny" or a "dope." None of the children were reported to idealize the therapist or have positive feelings toward him. What appears to have transpired in the treatment is that the therapist became the "bad" parent towards whom the child wanted to aggress. Unable to feel or direct hostility to his own parents or teachers, the unlovable therapist was a convenient target. This freed the youngster to function better in school, feel less depressed, and experience less hostility towards his actual parents. The therapist perhaps could have been regarded as that part of the parental introject who was beaten up and eventually killed off! It is quite conceivable that the children's experience with the therapist was subtly conveyed by the children to the parents, so that the latter got the message and moved away from "a love and be loved relationship" with their youngsters and limited them with more equanimity. (In two cases we have actual proof of this.)

Since the process described does not sound like a "cure" or complete working through or resolution of the child's ambivalence towards his parents, how are we to account for the youngsters' improved and sustained good functioning? Is it not possible to regard these children as relatively nondisturbed youngsters undergoing developmental hurdles in an environment which was not sufficiently supportive? As the youngsters moved toward more autonomy and separation, they experienced the movement as hostile attacks towards their "loving" parents. Unable to sincerely encourage expressions of assertiveness, separation, and autonomy, the parents unwillingly squelched the child's maturational movements and induced guilt and depression. The therapist, less narcissistically involved than the parents, could encourage the child to cathect negatively towards him and he thus provided an experience which the parents could not. Because the expression of anger was enjoyable to the child, he continued to retain this pleasure by saying in effect, "at least I don't have to love that therapist all the time; it's almost like hating my parents with impunity."

Implications

This report sheds some light on the parent-child relationships of some therapists. It would appear from our case material that most of these parents could be regarded as responsible, devoted and loving parents who were over-permissive and indulgent. Their inability to cope effectively with their childrens' aggression and assertiveness tended to freeze the youngsters in their interpersonal relationships. Perhaps therapists, out of their own feelings of "deprivation," tend to overgratify their children (and perhaps their patients, too?), which blocks assertive expressions and the growth process.

A therapist is someone the parents do not want to relate with on a close basis, but he is certainly somebody "who is good for the child." He offers the opportunity to help the child cope with his destructive wishes and to take on increasingly more frustration--so important for the growth process. Whether parents who are therapists are essentially different in their roles as parents from other middle-class occupational groups remains to be reported. However, it would seem that the availability of a therapist or similar figure can help certain children of therapists master the difficult developmental hurdles of autonomy and assertiveness.[2]

One of the significant implications emanating from the data is that some patients who leave treatment with an apparently negative transference, nevertheless have a good prognosis. Possibly similar to the parents under examination, who overtly championed a love and be loved relationship with their youngsters, many paychotherapists may regard successful psychotherapy as inherently dependent upon a positive transference and counter-transference relationship. It may well be important, however, for some patients to climb the psychosocial ladder successfully by leaving their therapists in anger or with negative feelings. If the therapist is experienced by the patient as part of an unnecessary symbiosis, as he appeared to be in several of the cases under examination, or as an unacceptable fragment of the patient's ego, terminating treatment with some significantly negative feeling toward the therapist may signify the beginning of healthy conflict resolution.

Notes

1. Alexander, R. and H. Ross. Dynamic Psychiatry. Chicago: University of Chicago Press, 1952, p. 8.

2. Erikson, E. Childhood and Society. New York: Norton, 1951.

3. Rosenblatt, A. The Application of Role Concepts to the Intake Process. Social Casework, Vol. XX, 1962.

4. Strean, H. The Use of the Patient as Consultant. Psychoanalysis and the Psychoanalytic Review, Vol. 46, No. 2, 1959.

5. Teicher, M. I. The Concept of Culture, Social Casework, Vol. XXX, 1958.

17. On Introducing the New Member

by Herbert S. Strean

From International Journal of Group Psychotherapy, vol. 12, no. 3, July 1962. Reprinted by permission.

It is virtually axiomatic in the theory and practice of group psychotherapy and group psychoanalysis that the advent of a new member in the group activates a complex interpersonal situation. Memories and affects related to siblings are stirred up, and ambivalent feelings toward the parents are reawakened. The therapeutic group, like any familial group, requires of its members and leader myriad adaptations at this point. Sub-groups become realigned, the parental surrogate has new demands made upon him, and the members, in turn, are obliged to relate to everyone in the group within a changed emotional constellation.

The purpose of this paper is to review, through the use of clinical illustrations, the multiple transference phenomena that were stimulated by the introduction of a new member into a group at different stages in the group's existence and development. The focus will be on an examination of the various stratagems utilized in introducing the new member and an evaluation of their relative merits.

The observations in this study were derived from a therapy group which met for three years, weekly, for an hour and a half, with the writer, at the Child Development Center in New York City. The Center is a therapeutic facility for the treatment of the preschool child and his family. Approximately five years ago the Center took note of the fact that, despite its philosophy of involving parents in a therapeutic program when their children were undergoing treatment, many fathers did not respond to invitations for therapy. Frequently, when they did, they were extremely resistant, feeling that: "This is part of the women's world and I don't belong." "I like to be an independent guy. I don't need you." "Who wants to be exposed and vulnerable? It's like being undressed." "I don't need a woman to tell me what to do." (Most of them had female therapists.) It was speculated that a group experience might be less threatening to these fathers, that they would not feel as exposed nor as vulnerable within an all-male group with the focus of attention diffused rather than limited to one individual.

Five fathers, all in their late thirties and early forties, business and professional men, attended the first twelve sessions. While their diagnoses varied, all showed characterological problems. The figure that dominated the early sessions was the enemy-therapist. He was a sinister individual who used "curious techniques to force people to talk against their will," "was concerned about money mostly," and "was for children and against parents." Each member in his own way brought out his distrust, disappointment, and discouragement with his previous therapeutic encounters. The group, as a unit, was clearly testing its current therapist.

With the program new and its success deeply desired, the therapist was eager to have Mr. J., a prospective candidate, join the fathers' group. After interviewing Mr. J. for three sessions, and carefully exploring his resistance, the therapist at the group's fourteenth session decided to broach the possibility of Mr. J.'s entrance to the group members (Ormont, 1957). Part of the session is reproduced verbatim:

> Leader: "There is the possibility of having a new member. How do you feel about it?" Mr. M. replies, "O.K. by me." After a silence, Mr. R. states, "I would like to know more about him. He's probably like one of us. A guy who can't get along with his kids." "Saw one of the women social workers and couldn't get along with her either," remarked Mr. T. All of the members and therapist laugh. Therapist asks what the laugh is about. Mr. Z. says, "Look, we're one big happy family, having a good time." Several members nod assent, and Mr. M. jocularly states, "That's why it's O.K. by me to have another guy. Maybe he'll help us knock those 'Lady Bountifuls'

> and we'll have an even better time." Mr. Z. turns to the leader and asks, "How do you feel about it?" The leader asks Mr. Z. and the group, how do they think the leader feels about this? Mr. Z. says, "You treat us pretty good so it'll probably help us." Exploration by the leader of the possibility of negative feelings toward the idea of a newcomer meets with either denial or silence. The group unanimously agrees that Mr. J. can be invited to the next meeting. One member summarizes, "He'll probably be a nice guy; without even meeting him I know it."

At the next session, Mr. J., the newcomer, was the first father to arrive, and the only one to arrive on time. Two members were absent for the first time: Mr. M., who had remarked it was O. K. by him to have a new member; and Mr. Z. who had seemed quite confident that a new member would enrich the group's spirit and morale. The theme of the session was "enlarging the members' families." En masse and without the therapist's intervention the men agreed that all of their families were complete, that their children would keenly resent a newcomer. Two of the fathers stated that they would not know how to talk to their children about this nor "handle their resistances." One father says, "A kid needs lots of preparation for this and he'll resent you if you don't help him. I suppose all kids hate their siblings at first but if the parent knows his business it'll work out." When the leader asked what it meant "if a parent knows his business," the response was, "He has to be clear why he wants the addition to the family and then he can cope with the kid's anger."

Although the members' discussion and behavior at this meeting is almost self-explanatory, it might be helpful to review more specifically its content as well as what transpired at the preceding session. As noted, the first twelve sessions involved heated discussions of the enemy-therapist. While the leader sensed that the members were testing him, he nonetheless continued to help them explore their negative feelings toward their previous female therapists. By the tone of the fourteenth session the members seemed to perceive him as a cheer leader supporting their negative feelings toward women. All hostility was directed toward the castrating women, and the therapist was consciously experienced as a lovable guy. One must ask, how much gratification was this offering to the therapist? How competitive was he with the patient's previous therapists? How accurate was one member's perception when he implied that the leader was bringing in the new member so that 'Lady Bountifuls' could be knocked?

The therapist's unconscious fear of the members' hostility is suggested by his tentative question, "There is the possibility of having a new member. How do you feel about it?" Permissive, tentative, ingratiatory, he prohibited the expression of negative feelings. The group overtly stated that they wanted the newcomer to join the group and all seemed quite "comfy". However, two members absented themselves from the next meeting and three arrived late. Through their children they really say, "This group is complete, Mr. Therapist, but you don't realize it! We resent the newcomer; you did not prepare us, and you did not handle our resistances. We needed a lot more preparation and you don't know your business. You have to be clear about your motives and learn to cope with our hostility."

In succeeding sessions the members were helped to bring out their anger toward the therapist, likened him to their previous therapists, and recalled memories revolving around the arrival of younger siblings. The advent of the newcomer to the fathers' group and the ldeader's handling of the situation was eventually seen as the event that precipitated negative feelings toward the therapist and the recollection of old and unpleasant memories.

The group turned, in later sessions, to their feelings of incompetence in their work and their inadequacy as men. Feelings of competition toward each other and the leader emerged. Fear of reprisal after ventilation of aggression was a conflict shared by most members and it was thoroughly investigated. The group transference shifted and the leader was seen more frequently as the strong, powerful father and occasionally as the omnipotent, gratifying, but occasionally begrudging mother.

Six members attended the meetings faithfully for close to a year. In the fall of the second year, after the group met for three sessions, another member was introduced. A partial account of the forty-fifth session is presented:

> Leader: "I am planning to bring in a new member soon" (A one-minute silence). Mr. M. says, "Ah nuts, we're doing fine without one. It's tough enough listening to five guys. Another one, I'm against it." Mr. Z. answers, "Well, let's be fair. I wouldn't like to be rejected. Maybe he's a nice guy. Why should we keep him out!" Remarks Mr. T., "Well, I'm not sure it's up to us. Strean said he's planning to bring in a new member. He didn't ask our permission." Two members nod in agreement and another father says, "You are getting tougher on us. So it's <u>not</u> up to us!" Several members rally and tell the therapist that if they had no say in the matter, maybe the group shouldn't discuss it. Mr. Z. recalls how his father moved from one city to another when he, Mr. Z., was five and to this day he resents his father for it. Mr. M. responds by bellowing, "I resent the group leader acting like a big shot. Is it his group or ours?"

In succeeding sessions, with the newcomer's arrival still in doubt as far as the members were concerned, the fathers discussed their feelings of impotence and inferiority in relation to their own fathers. "A strong confident father helps a boy in liking his own masculinity." Three fathers talked about their resentment toward their own fathers because they weren't sufficiently decisive. "Too much was on my shoulders and it wasn't good." Mr. Z. recalled how the last time a new member was introduced, the storm took place afterwards. "It's better this time. We are getting it out. But you keep us dangling." When the leader stated that the new member would be coming in the next week or two, the members seemed a little relieved and each in his own way said, "At last! But we still don't know for sure <u>when</u>."

When the newcomer arrived, after a few pleasantries, the theme of the discussion without intervention on the therapist's part was: "Waiting at the hospital until the wife delivers." The members all felt that this was an extremely anxiety-provoking situation filled with eagerness and pleasure but coupled with apprehension and fantasies of possible damage to the child. "Will it be a boy or a girl and what will it turn out to be?"

In further sessions the men discussed their feelings about a newcomer arriving on the job. A threat to their own status, a possible usurping of their roles, and a change in staff relationships were mentioned and discussed. Change always induces anxiety, the men agreed, and all people have their own ways of dealing with it. Memories of sibling arrivals were again revived, with the majority of the men agreeing, "If my parents really loved me, why did they have another?" Eventually they saw their reactions as being provoked by the leader's introduction of the new member. The men were clearly ambivalent in their feelings toward the new member and the leader.

In this second example, there was a more genuine expression of feelings prior to the newcomer's arrival. The group saw the leader as a stronger father but yet, how strong he was, was not certain. They recalled resenting their own fathers for being indecisive and wished that their fathers had made decisions more promptly. The therapist's wavering about the date of the arrival of the newcomer provoked these memories and the members felt quite ambivalent toward him. It is his plan this time and this permitted a ventilation of aggression on the spot. But, who is the boss and what is the status of each member in the group remained in doubt. "If the therapist really loved his symbolic family, would he do this?" seemed to be one of the major themes.

We have reviewed two instances of a new member being introduced to a group at different stages in its development. When a new member was introduced in the first example, the leader appeared uncertain, insecure, and ingratiating. This provoked the members to consider their roles as leaders of their own families and precipitated a discussion of their own uncertainty and insecurity in adding a new member to their current families. It further activated memories of a new sibling entering their original families and helped the men recapture memories when their own parents behaved with uncertainty and insecurity. The group members could relive traumas of being unprepared to face crucial life events after they directed their anger at the therapist. That anxiety and trauma were mastered is demonstrated by their turning to a consideration of their roles as men. They were able to expose problems of anxiety on the job, for example. Consequently, we can fairly safely conclude that regardless of the leader's reasons and motivations for his tentativeness, ingratiation, and uncertainty, the experiences in the group which followed his mentioning a new member were therapeutic.

At the time of the second introduction, the group themes had oedipal overtones; competition, strength, and status were group preoccupations, and the group transference toward the therapist was more on an oedipal level. Here, the leader on introducing the new member appeared more confident and certain of his role. It is his plan this time and it induced the group to question, who is boss around here? The father as an ego ideal emerged as a consideration, and memories relating to father's strength or lack of strength, his decisiveness or dilly-dallying, were of concern to the members. When the leader did not state the date the new member was going to arrive, the members recalled memories of waiting for the baby to arrive and similar life events where the future is not exactly known. The close-to-universal feeling that, "If mommy and daddy really loved me, they would not have had another child," is related to the transference feeling, "If you, Mr. Therapist, really love us, why do you increase the size of the group?"

Again, we must state that regardless of the therapist's reasons for his method of introduction, the therapeutic sessions were rich, dynamic, and unraveled important memories.

My experiences with this fathers' group and other groups, as well as my discussions with other group therapists on introducing the new member have prompted a total reconsideration of this important event in a group's life, and a model for introducing a new member into any therapeutic group has evolved.

Kaplan and Roman (1961) concluded that the introduction of a new member into adult groups provoked a trauma for its members. They likened the characteristic responses of the adult group members to children attempting to master anxiety through play. Regression is induced by introducing a new member, and the writers imply that the therapist must play the right game at the right time.

To play the right game at the right time is a difficult

task. To help with this, paradigmatic psychotherapy, introduced by Coleman and Nelson in 1956, may shed some light. The paradigmatic therapist first attempts to understand as well as possible his patient or patients. He identifies the resistances, transferences, and group themes, and then elects a role which will stimulate the most productive affective expression of repressed conflict. He may join resistances, reduplicate introjected images, mirror unrecognized behavior, or use other stratagems which help the patient recognize what he feels rather than why he feels. He attempts to ascertain what is the game the patient is playing, what childhood event or events is he recapitulating, and then chooses the correct role for the game so that the psychological trauma may be re-enacted in the therapeutic arena rather than remain dormant, intellectually interpreted, or acted out.

What is the best role for a group therapist to select on introducing a new member to a group? If we liken this event to introducing an infant to a family, we may find it. To have a baby is the parents' decision. *They* plan for the child and only *they* can reproduce it. When conception takes place, *they* decide when to tell the rest of the family of *their* decision. They tell their children approximately when the baby is coming, but what he or she will be like, no one can foretell. The sex, the size, the shape are mysteries. That the children are entitled to have a response is beyond question. They can fantasy what they would like or not like to have. They have a right to express what it means to them, and parents have an obligation to prepare the children, absorb their children's feelings, and encourage their expression. But it is their baby and when it comes, family members need help in adapting to the event, and new roles, tasks, and assignments must be constantly considered and examined (Strean, 1960).

Using the birth process as our model, the birth is the game the group therapist should play. He should assume the role of the parent who decides when the family is ready for the newcomer. He produces the child, but at which group session is his decision, not the group's. He can tell them approximately the session the new member is coming, but precisely which one should be a surprise. He does not announce the sex, shape, or size of the newcomer but welcomes fantasies about the newcomer and encourages the expression of feelings and wishes concerning the event. He certainly prepares the group, not by giving information about the newcomer but by welcoming reactions to the members' interpretation of the event. When the newcomer arrives, he reassesses his group, attempts to understand how the group family is doing--who is the big brother, who is the displaced sibling, who is the jealous child competing with the parent--and then elects a new role which will enable the modified family to live on.

In conclusion, although the model of the birth process is constantly borne in mind in introducing the new member, the therapist's role has to be adapted to the group's development, group transference, group themes, and group resistances.

References

Coleman, M. and Nelson, B. (1957), Paradigmatic Psychotherapy in Borderline Treatment. Psychoanalysis, 5:28-44.

Kaplan, S.R., and Roman, M. (1961), Characteristic Responses in Adult Therapy to the Introduction of New Members: A Reflection of Group Processes. This Journal, 11:372-381.

Ormont, L.R. (1957), The Preparation of Patients for Group Psychoanalysis. Am. J. Psychother., 11:841-848.

Strean, H. (1960), Treating Parents of Emotionally Disturbed Children Through Role Playing. Psychoanal. & Psychoanal. Rev., 47:67-75.

Part III

Family Treatment

18. A Means of Involving Fathers in Family Treatment: Guidance Groups for Fathers

by Herbert S. Strean

From The American Journal of Orthopsychiatry, vol. 32, no. 4, July 1962. Reprinted by permission.

The role of the father in our society has been difficult to grasp. As customs, beliefs, thought, and knowledge change, the father's role assumes new forms.

Our Victorian stereotype of the distant, taciturn, and stern father has been undergoing modification. The more modern picture of the father is that of a gregarious young man interested in his wife and children, who likes his home and likes to work around it. He enjoys helping his wife with household duties and with the routine of child care. (3).

We should like to believe that our current conception of the modern father is a realistic one, and that he is replacing the older types. Unfortunately, facts seem to show that society in general, and fathers in particular, find it extremely difficult to define the role of the contemporary father (1, p. 63).

Of the many institutions in our society that have changed their perspective on the father's participation in the family, mental hygiene clinics, family agencies, and child guidance clinics are among the most prominent. In contrast to earlier years, when clinics and social agencies tended to work largely with the mother, or with the mother and child, there is evidence that a new trend is in operation. Currently, an attempt is being made to involve more and more fathers in various types of treatment procedures (2).

While the literature is replete with case examples showing the soundness of various treatment methods as they pertain to fathers, to this writer's knowledge few attempts have been made to describe the processes inherent in the simultaneous treatment of several fathers in a guidance group.[1]

The aim in a guidance group is to increase the parent's adequacy of functioning in his day-to-day relationship with the child. Theoretically, this aim is achieved by involving fathers in a group where discussion is held mainly on father-child relationships and father-child conflicts.

This paper, therefore, will deal with the writer's experience in treating several fathers through the medium of a guidance group. The question to be answered is: Do guidance groups help fathers, and, if so, how do they help create a more favorable family climate for their members?

In attempting to examine the writer's experience with this group, several areas will be investigated: 1) the group composition--the men themselves, their backgrounds, their families, their motivations for joining the group; 2) content of the sessions--what the fathers talked about, how they related to each other and to the therapist; and 3) an attempt by the therapist to demonstrate how he related to the material brought out in the sessions.

The group met at the Madeleine Borg Child Guidance Institute of the Jewish Board of Guardians for a little over a year. The men met once every two weeks in the evening for an hour and a half and participated in approximately 20 sessions.

When the group was initiated in January 1957, it consisted of six men. Each was the father of two children, of whom at least one had been in treatment from two to three years. The wives of all of the men had been in treatment for approximately the same length of time as the children.

In June 1957, two fathers already in individual treatment joined the group and the membership than totaled eight. The attendance at meetings, however, remained around five.

Most of these men were described by intake workers as passive, weak, defeated fathers, but they were very strongly resistant to treatment for themselves. They felt that the wife made the major decisions, particularly in the area of child rearing. They, the fathers, did not have time for, or interest in, getting involved with the agency. It seemed equivalent to invading the women's world, of which they wanted no part. At intake they frequently provoked rejection or hostility and emerged as outsiders in the treatment of their families. It is important to emphasize that these very fathers, who were described as passive, weak and not very active in participating in their own families, became in each case nonparticipants in the treatment of their respective families.

> The case of Mr. A provides a good illustration. A mild but constant depreciator of his wife and children's behavior, Mr. A's major contributions to the family were his salary and an occasional exhibition of his athletic prowess to his daughters. He delegated all family decisions and child rearing to Mrs. A. Resentful of Mr. A's disinterest and apathy, she felt compelled to fill the vacuum left by her husband. Though there were constant arguments between the parents over Mr. A's emotional isolation, the mother consistently ruled with an iron hand and the father nodded to her decisions.
>
> The A children's reactive behavior disorders complicated the tenuous family balance and their hyperactive and frequently contemptuous behavior only added insult to the injurious family relationships.
>
> Though against psychotherapy, Mr. A apprehensively went along with Mrs. A's initiation of treatment for their daughters. Mr. A came for only one intake interview during the two years his "three girls" (wife and two daughters) were in treatment. This family situation is quite typical of many under discussion.

Though united in their resistance against treatment, the fathers in the group varied widely in occupations and in family constellations. Among them were a commercial artist, a jewelry-store owner, a mailman, a salesman, and the owner of a religious goods store. Most of the fathers were in their forties, and their children ranged in age from 3 to 20 years.

As indicated, all of these fathers were threatened by the prospect of treatment for themselves but responded to the idea of a guidance group. Why should this happen? To answer this question, some of the men's comments may serve as a clue. "If I want to talk, I can talk. If I want to listen, I listen. If I want to shut up, I shut up" . . . "What a good way to get away from the wife and kids for the night, smoke a cigar and relax" . . . "It's always good to know that other guys have troubles too" . . . "I wanted to be part of the plan here but they weren't too eager to have me" . . . "In a group you won't get to that unconscious stuff" . . . "It's good to be with men and men only."

It seemed then that the idea of group treatment was less disturbing to these men than individual treatment. The fear of having their own pathology explored was allayed. The opportunity to discuss universal problems and to leave their children for an evening was a possible reason for the unanimous response to the idea of a group. Evidently, too, the guidance group was perceived by some as a further opportunity to insulate themselves from the rest of the family.

It should be mentioned that the group therapist had several ideas in mind when interviewing all the prospective members individually. The group was presented as strictly voluntary and experimental, and each individual's defensive structure was supported. The man reluctant to talk in groups was told that we would be interested in evaluating what the group could offer to one who remained solely a listener. The father who bragged about how he handled his son skillfully was told that here might be an opportunity to be an advice-giver. The men were further told that we would be talking about father-child relationships principally and would not be directly concerned with marriage, in-laws, etc.

Of the men available as potential candidates for the guidance group, none could be described as overtly destructive in the family constellation. On the contrary, they seemed psychologically unavailable as fathers and unavailable as treatment candidates.

In reviewing the first four or five sessions of the group, we found that the continual theme appeared to be how tough it is to be a father and how much more fun it is to be a child. The fathers all agreed that the demands placed on them were enormous and extremely difficult if not impossible to fulfill. The following were typical reactions to their children's demands: "I have to give him more money for an allowance than I ever got" . . . "They keep wanting to watch television all the time and I never get my turn" . . . "If you give one kid attention, the other one hollers, so you quit after awhile" . . . "It's too much. You'd think they'd realize that I had a hard day and I'm entitled to some rest."

The men drew a strong contrast between the way children in this generation seek to be indulged and the firm and punitive way the fathers themselves had been handled by their own parents. The memory of the "lockshen strap"[2] was revived on more than one occasion.

When the members were confronted with the fact that from time to time children need limits and are capable of arousing legitimate and honest anger in adults, most members of the group expressed great surprise. Defensive maneuvers were erected to protect themselves from seeing children any differently. "He's my child; I have to love him and give him everything," said one father.

Although the therapist tried very hard to support the defenses and resistances of the fathers by allowing them to express resentment about their burdens, and although he suggested that they did not have to meet every one of their children's demands, he was still seen as an ungiving person. He was attacked for not giving more information on techniques in child rearing. He was told that he was too withdrawn and passive a person, and it was suggested that perhaps he could serve the men beer or cookies and coffee.

Evidently these fathers wanted to be fed more than the therapist was feeding them. Though they complained bitterly that their children made too many demands on them, which they felt incapable of meeting, they put themselves in exactly the same demanding position in regard to the therapist. Their behavior in the group was certainly in many instances a repetition of their children's behavior at home.

> Mr. A, a humorous depreciator of his wife's interaction with the children, made fun of events that other fathers described. Mr. T, a self-righteous

moralist who insisted on adult-like behavior from his son, frowned upon any display of regression in the group. Mr. S, a very provocative man in his relationship with his son, aroused so much hostility in the other men that they tried their best to get him to withdraw from the group. His methods of withdrawal from the group were very similar to those he used in withdrawing psychologically from his own home. Finally, Mr. L, who was Mother's Little Helper at home, always insisted on helping the therapist in as many ways as he could find.

It can be concluded that the group was for many of its members a symbolic family. The men used each other and the therapist to act out neurotic problems in old and current relationships. Though the men obviously protected themselves from freely interacting with each other by various defensive maneuvers, their need to establish themselves as members of a symbolic family was ever-present.

Frequently the therapist emerged as the object to cathect unresolved problems. He might be loved and hated as were the members' parents or siblings in the past. For example, at about the sixth session when the men were beginning to report some changes--"giving my son what he needs rather than what he wants" . . . "allowing myself to be really annoyed at my daughter and not feeling so guilty afterwards"--they openly attacked the therapist for being incompetent.

When the therapist asked what was wrong with him and why they thought he was a poor therapist, the men said he made them work too hard, that he did not supply solutions to perplexing questions, or give them enough theoretical data. This experience of seeing the therapist subject the members' complaints to examination turned out to be a key session and changed the tone of the next several meetings. The fathers began to acknowledge openly in the group their own personal limitations as people, as husbands, and as fathers. They started to allow themselves to admit directly personal as well as interpersonal problems.

It is suggested that when the therapist allows himself to be subjected to examination, the group members will eventually subject themselves to a similar examination.

Typical statements made by the fathers after the session referred to above are the following: "I asked my son what is going on between us since we can't get along very well and we had a great discussion" . . . "Johnny wasn't going to bed on time and there was a fight every night. I looked at myself and saw that I really wanted him to stay up."

Whether a group therapist allows himself to be subjected to examination or not, inevitably he will be. The nature of a therapeutic group is such that the group will respond to the therapist's unconscious. At the seventh session, when the therapist's position in the agency was in doubt, the group chose to discuss separation anxiety.

At about the thirteenth session, the therapist out of his own needs called a very early meeting right after Labor Day. The men spent most of their time talking about their hard-working youthful days and competed to see who got paid the least.

It was interesting too that, after one of these sessions, a father exclaimed: "Sometimes kids know exactly what's on your mind. You don't even have to say anything; they pick up the subtleties."

Although the group was structured to discuss solely parent-child conflicts, they began to discuss marital problems, conflicts with their own parents, and in-laws. Actually this evolved very interestingly. After criticizing their children, they attacked and criticized the therapist. Next they criticized their wives, then each other and finally themselves. This changed the classic structure of the traditional guidance group. Under the stimulation of the psychiatric consultant for this group, and with the group therapy consultant concurring, it was decided to let the group be an arena for all feelings in all relationships instead of limiting discussions to parent-child relationships.

Coupled with a growing open ventilation of individual problems were various attempts to test the therapist. The members wanted to see if he was really honest in his convictions. Around the fourteenth session, after the therapist had supported statements of the members regarding the importance of their own individual pleasures, and they had begun to limit their children appropriately, they started to dawdle and stay beyond the time allotted for the meetings. When the therapist was forced to say that he wanted to go home and relax because he had had a hard day, the fathers were quite impressed and later gave examples of having allowed themselves to "take it easy" at home.

Another phenomenon which seemed to evolve in this group was a developmental scheme. During the early sessions there was much discussion on oral problems such as thumb-sucking and excessive eating. After a while discussion turned to anal problems: toilet-training, problems of controlling, saving and withholding.

Not only were oral and anal problems discussed as such, but the men's behavior toward each other and toward the therapist showed what level they were operating on. Still later, phallic and genital problems were discussed, such as masturbation and sexual relations. The discussions in the group went back and forth without giving the therapist much opportunity to predict what would happen next.

This developmental sequence offers us another clue to the members' perception of the group. Frequently the group fosters growing up. Having demanded to be "fed," the members in turn often "fed" the surrogate parent by developing better controls and demonstrating more mature behavior. After this type of experience, the men should be in a better position to help their own children develop.

Perhaps, at this point, an attempt can be made to answer the question: "Do guidance groups help fathers, and if so, how do they provide a better family climate for their members?"

To the first part of the question, "Do guidance groups help fathers?" the writer's answer is "yes and no." There are men who have attended group meetings very infrequently and they have provided much information on some of the negative aspects of a guidance group.

One man said, "You don't talk enough about wives; that's my problem--I've got to get that fixed up." This man is being helped toward individual treatment and perhaps that is what should have occurred in the first place. Another father said, "I don't like all men in groups. We need women in here, too." In other words, a fathers' group may arouse in some men so much homosexual anxiety that they withdraw. Moreover some men find more aggression than they can tolerate; they become panicky and also withdraw.

In a fathers' group the major focus is on guidance, although in the group described this was somewhat modified. To some men discussion in this medium does not affect underlying pathology sufficiently and hence their relationships at home are not altered appreciably.

On the positive side, a guidance group for fathers can provide a sympathetic male audience. This can offer strength, understanding, and support. New techniques on child rearing are picked up, tried and often integrated. A guidance group offers members the opportunity to feel "I'm not so alone in this world; other guys have troubles too." Offered a chance to regress in the group, they often show mature behavior on the outside. After one member had brought out a tremendous amount of hostility toward his wife and daughters, which was subjected to considerable analysis in the group, he asked his wife, "How can I learn to understand you better?"

Many fathers who are outsiders in the family, if offered an opportunity to participate in the treatment plan, can mobilize a greater willingness to participate as members of their own families. Participation in a symbolic family can pave the way for participation in a real family.

The aim in a guidance group is to increase the parents' adequacy of functioning in the day-to-day relationship with their children. While there is some evidence that the children often react positively when the father is increasingly sensitized to their needs, further collaboration is needed with the workers treating other members of the family. It is important to have more impressions and observations of the advantages and disadvantages that accrue after a father enters a guidance group.

All too frequently a child guidance clinic or family agency is confronted with a strong, seemingly powerful, controlling mother and a threatened, weak, passive, defeated father. Fearful of treatment for himself, the father retires once more and becomes a withdrawn outsider. A guidance group may be a means of uniting him with his family, giving him some strength to cope with the burdens of being a parent, and helping him to enjoy some of its potential pleasures.

Notes

1. S. R. Slavson introduced the procedure of guidance groups for parents. The background of his work is described in a recent book (4).
2. A strap with appendages at the end, traditionally used by many European Jewish families to punish children.

References

1. Burgess, Ernest W., and Harvey J. Locke. The Family. Chicago: American Book Co., 1947.
2. Editorial Notes. Soc. Casewk., 35:354-355, 1954.
3. English, O. Spurgeon. The Psychological Role of the Father in the Family. Casewk., 35:323-329, 1954.
4. Slavson, Samuel R. Child-Centered Group Guidance of Parents. New York: Internat. Univ. Press, 1958.

19. Non-Verbal Cues and Reenactment of Conflict in Family Therapy

by Murray H. Sherman,
Nathan W. Ackerman,
Sanford N. Sherman, and
Celia Mitchell

From *Family Process*, vol. 4, no. 1., March 1965. Reprinted by permission. Originally, the authors noted that their "acknowledgement and thanks are offered to the entire professional staff of the Family Mental Health Clinic of the Jewish Family Service of New York, whose thoughtful suggestions and critical comments have been incorporated in this paper."

When the entire family is seen together in therapy, there is the opportunity to observe a reenactment of the specific conflict which has brought the family to treatment (1). This enactment of conflict is attributable to many factors, among which is the family's need to demonstrate their emotional turmoil to the therapist in order to gain his help in resolving the family neurosis. However, the family conflict also has a static, perseverative quality which leads to its continuance in all sorts of situations in and out of treatment. One of the major advantages of family therapy is the opportunity afforded the therapist to observe and intervene in these perseverative enactments *in situ*, on the very scene of battle.

Within any given session it is often difficult to detect the specific origins of a particular conflict enactment at the very moment it is occurring. These origins are doubtless of a multidimensional sort, but among them the significance of non-verbal cues has been noted with increasing frequency (5, 9). As a matter of fact, the significance of such subtleties of non-verbal communication as tonal inflections and fleeting facial expressions has long been noted as characteristic of the psychoanalytic situation (8, 10, 11), but only now are these data being explored in a systematic, scientic fashion. The development of such scientific recording devices as the tape recorder and motion picture camera has undoubtedly been a major factor in the study of fleeting aspects of non-verbal expressions. The scientific description of the startle pattern (6) and its diagnostic significance was made possible by examination of individual frames of motion picture recording.

The traditional role of the psychotherapist has tended to include relatively less attention to these non-verbal behaviors than to the verbal content that is communicated. Moreover, the specific relationships between non-verbal cues and the psychodynamics of family conflict have not yet been demonstrated in detail with illustrative case material. The problems of this type of study have been explored from the standpoints of kinesics (4) and of paralinguistic analysis (7), but our intent here is to deal with more molar cues that could be detected in ordinary therapeutic interaction, were the therapist to pay particular heed to these minute behavioral expressions.

The basic therapeutic data are exceedingly hard come by. It is only too well known that a therapist's own report of his sessions will often omit much of the most vital interaction, even where there is a sincere effort to communicate this material. Tape recordings lose much of the subtle interaction and communication of therapy, and non-verbal cues are often totally missed in taped transcriptions. Sound films are undoubtedly the most satisfactory form of recording of both verbal and non-verbal behavior, despite the almost prohibitive expense involved. Even these sound films require transcription if they are to be scientifically analyzed, and the transcription, if conscientiously done, is a most time consuming task.

One gets the impression that something is transpiring in the therapeutic process which has almost its own resistance to deeper understanding. There seems to be an exceedingly subtle intercommunication that transpires at a very basic and even primitive level, and this process somehow eludes us when we try to translate it into verbal form.

An almost transcendent, secretive quality becomes attached to the subtleties of a therapeutic relationship, which defies even the most searching and strenuous efforts at explicit description. It seems likely that non-verbal cues do play a most significant role in this tenuous process and a detailed investigation of their functions in the re-enactment of family conflict may cast some light upon the more general problem of therapeutic communication.

The B Family

It was decided to investigate a filmed sample of non-verbal behavior as this emerged within the context of family therapy. We were interested both in the therapeutic use that could be made of non-verbal behavior and also in the specific forms in which this behavior reflected the total family conflict.

The B. family was chosen for this investigation because a preliminary viewing of a sound film of one of their family therapy sessions indicated a plentitude of non-verbal behavior.

The B. family consisted of Mr. Jack B., aged 52, whose occupation was that of half-owner of a hardward business;[1] Mrs. Joan B., aged 43 and a school teacher; Sam, aged 16; and Ann, aged 10. (Names and other identifying data have been disguised.) The incident precipitating this family's coming to the clinic occurred about two months prior to the filmed session. Ann had become very angry and excited and had gone into a temper tantrum in which she had taken a large knife and threatened Sam with it. Sam was overcome by a fit of fear, ran into his parents' bedroom to tell them what was happening and had then apparently collapsed on the bed in a cold, perspiring faint.

This incident was the culmination of a long series of conflicts in which Ann had continually intimidated and manipulated the entire family. Mrs. B. was almost totally unable to discipline Ann and would resort to various manipulative strategems to make her eat or behave as she should; these strategems were admittedly ineffective. Mrs. B. would then make periodic efforts to draw up lists of preemptory rules of family behavior, which were soon ignored. Mrs. B. attributed her inability to discipline Ann to her relationship with her own mother, whom she described as overbearing, overprotective and highly demanding. Mrs. B.'s own father was described as passive and ineffectual; she called him a "horror," a term which she also applied to Sam as a difficult infant.

Sam's relation with his mother was a highly ambivalent and inconsistent one. Mrs. B. was overly solicitous about Sam's health and he would resent this and withdraw from it. On the other hand, when Mrs. B. got angry with Sam, he would become very disturbed, would reassure his mother that he loved her very much and plead that she not be angry with him.

Mr. B.'s parents had been divorced when he was seven, and he had lived with his mother who tried to encourage him to be "independent." In his own marriage Mr. B.'s work often kept him away overnight, and he generally took a passive and unassertive role. A particular incident well illustrates the lines of control and interaction in this family. Ann had become angry with Sam and wanted to poke him in retaliation for something he had done. She asked her parents each to hold one of Sam's arms so she could poke him. Mr. B. refused to do this but stood by as Mrs. B. held both of Sam's arms, and Ann obtained her revenge.

For several years prior to coming to therapy at the agency Mrs. B. had had a severe case of torticollis and had consulted a number of psychiatrists and other medical specialists. She had finally been cured by massive injections (nature undetermined) and used this as evidence that there had been no psychological meaning to the symptoms. Sam's symptomatic picture included a bizarre masturbatory ritual in which he would telephone hospitals and ask them for information on how to feed a resistant infant. Sam would provoke his informant into telling him to use force if necessary, and this was highly exciting to him.

There is an interesting confluence of symptoms among the three generations. Mrs. B.'s own mother had had the habit of continually passing wind. Mrs. B.'s belching, as will be evident in the session below, was a highly significant aspect of her relationship to her husband. Sam, when emotionally disturbed, was prone to vomit. All three individuals apparently converted their aggression into an involuntary eruption through a bodily orifice.

The B. family was seen in family therapy by a caseworker over a period of one year and there were also periodic interviews (eight) by Dr. A. Ann's behavior became much improved. She was more controlled and the temper tantrums receded. Mrs. B.'s preoccupation with Ann's eating habits also receded but was replaced by an obsession with her school work. On one occasion Mrs. B. so annoyed Ann by inquiring whether she had done her homework that Ann deliberately tore it to shreds before her mother's eyes.

There was some active inquiry and handling of the sexual relationship between Mr. and Mrs. B. Mr. B. complained that his wife was not active enough in sex and said that he felt certain wives could learn a good deal from prostitutes, whom he had known before marriage. Mrs. B. complained that her husband was an inadequate lover and did not satisfy her. She said that his demands, if she acceded to them, would make sex much too mechanical for her. During the course of therapy Mr. B. became more active in sex, but there was not a great deal of improvement.

Family therapy was hindered by a number of resistances which developed. When anger was expressed by the children during the session, Mrs. B. felt that this was very bad because it was just what she was coming to therapy to prevent. Mr. B. objected to the explicitness of sexual discussion. Various family members would become ill, which prevented the family's being seen together. There were also fee difficulties; the parents felt the fee was too high and they were frequently behind in payments. Nevertheless, despite all these difficulties, it was felt that therapy had made certain significant gains and that much had been accomplished in family understanding and improved relationships.

A Family Therapy Session

In order to develop the accompanying transcript of a sound film of family therapy, a tape recording was made from which the dialogue was taken. Then the film itself was watched approximately one dozen times to fill in the visual and other contexts. Many minute aspects of family communication, such as subtle facial expressions and small bodily movements, have nevertheless been lost, despite considerable effort to include some of the most essential and noticeable ones. One wonders whether the return from such effort merely to transcribe and communicate yields a commensurate reward. On the other hand, the very difficulty of this task leads one to believe that a special secret must somehow be buried in these mountains of words and gestures.

Transcript of Sound Film

1. Dr.: Jack, you heaved a sigh as you sat down.
2. Mr. B.: Just physical, not mental.
3. Dr.: Whom are you kidding?
4. Mr. B.: Kidding no one.
5. Dr.: (warningly) Jack!
6. Mr. B.: I'm tired because I put in a full day.
7. Dr.: Well, I'm tired every day. When I sigh, it's never purely physical.
8. Mr. B.: Really?
9. Dr.: Yes. What's the matter?
10. Mr. B.: Nothing. Really.
11. Sam: (laughs)
12. Dr.: Your own son doesn't believe that.
13. Mr. B.: Well, I mean nothing, nothing caused me to sigh specially today, or tonight.
14. Dr.: Well, maybe it isn't so special, but--uh-- How about it, Sam?
15. Sam: (shakes head no)
16. Dr.: You wouldn't know? All of a sudden you put on a poker face. You do it very knowingly.
17. Mr. B.: (laughs)
18. Sam: I really don't know.
19. Dr.: Well, do you know anything about your Pop?
20. Sam: Yeah.
21. Dr.: What do you know about him?
22. Sam: Well, I don't know except that I know something about him.
23. Dr.: Well, let's hear.
24. Sam: Well, I (laughs nervously)--he's a man.
25. Dr.: He's a man?
26. Mr. B.: (makes beckoning gesture with his hand to Sam) Come on, come on, Dr. A. wants some

information from you.

27\. Sam: All right, I'll tell you Dr. A.

28\. Dr.: Your father uses his hand (referring to beckoning gesture), you know. Not like mother. She has another gesture. Give, give, give (demonstrates). Mother's gesture is this (shows). Pop's gesture is give (Father laughing loudly all this while.)

29\. Sam: I don't have much to say about Dad. He's just a normal man. He's my father. He's a good guy, that's all.

30\. Mrs. B.: May I make a suggestion?

31\. Dr.: What's your suggestion?

32\. Mrs. B.: Well, I have been keeping an anecdotal record of the time that has elapsed since we were here. Not every minute of the time, but anything that I think is important enough to relate. Now, I think this is good for many reasons. When you read, you sort of get a better view of things, and if you'd like me to read it, I will. If you feel you'd rather ask question, you can. But--uh--that's my suggestion.

33\. Dr.: Well, I'm glad you called my attention to that notebook that's in your lap. You come armed with a notebook, a record.

34\. Mrs. B.: I've been doing this in school, as a matter of fact.

35\. Dr.: I see.

36\. Mrs. B.: And I've been keeping this record since last week, because I think it's very important. You forget very quickly what people say and how they say it, unless you write it down right away. Now, this is something that I do for children in the class that I have to have their case histories. And I think it's a wonderful idea.

37\. Dr.: Well now, what have you there? A case history on your whole family?

38\. Mrs. B.: Yes

39\. Dr.: Marvelous! How long is it?

40\. Mrs. B.: It's not that long. I just started it. (Jack starts to read over Joan's shoulder.) There's something here that you didn't see last night.

41\. Mr. B.: Oh, you cheated!

42\. Mrs. B.: I didn't cheat. I just didn't tell you there was more.

43. Mr. B.: That's cheating.

44. Mrs. B.: No, it isn't. So, if you would like me to read it. It's sort of a little resume of my thinking in the last week. I was quite disturbed last week in the middle of the week, very disturbed. So much so that on the last day of school, a little girl in my class gave me a pin, a four leaf clover pin. Now I never told this little girl anything. She said, "Maybe this will change your luck." So I was very disturbed and that's what made me do this. I felt it's better to come with exact words and phrases rather than remembering things.

45. Dr.: Now--uh--is this a four leaf clover? Is that what you've got?

46. Mrs. B.: Yes.

47. Dr.: That change your luck?

48. Mrs. B.: No, not yet it hasn't, but--

49. Dr.: Have you got it on you?

50. Mrs. B.: No. I didn't wear it tonight but it was very sweet and I, I cried for a little while after she left, because I was so--

51. (Mr. B. picks at his finger and Dr. notices.)

52. Dr.: Your finger hurting?

53. Mr. B.: No, I was--had a little hangnail.

54. Mrs. B.: That's a nervous ailment of his. He picks at his feet, at a rash there and he picks at his fingers. That's a nervous ailment of *his*.

55. Sam: Pretty disgusting (laughs amusedly).

56. Dr.: Pretty disgusting, is it?

57. Sam: (to mother) What about your nervous habits?

58. Mrs. B.: I have quite a few.

59. Sam: Like sitting and--never mind. Quite a few.

60. Mrs. B.: I said I have a few.

61. Sam: Yeah, and they're pretty bad, because when I--

62. Dr.: Are you sore at mother because she's picking pieces out of Papa's uh--

63. Sam: Yeah.

64. Dr.: Fingers?

65. Sam: Yeah; so what? So he has nervous habits. So don't we all?

66. Dr.: What kind of a piece would you pick, like to pick out of Mama?

67. Sam: Huh? She has some pretty disgusting habits.
68. Dr.: Well, what are they?
69. Mrs. B.: I'll tell you what they are.
70. Dr.: Now wait a minute. Sam is talking.
71. Sam: Uh--(laughs nervously).
72. Mrs. B.: Well, Sam, you don't have to be bashful. This is to give information. You don't have to be--
73. Dr.: He's not bashful.
74. Mrs. B.: --embarrassed, in my mind.
75. Dr.: Hold it, hold it, hold it. Now, Sam.
76. Sam: I don't know how to put it, if you want the truth.
77. Mrs. B.: That's why I was going to put it for you.
78. Sam: Yeah, well I, maybe she has some better words for the thing.
79. Dr.: No, no, no, no, now. This is, is that same old give, Sam, here to me (repeat father's gesture as above), the same old insincere ritual, you first Alphonse. Let's not be scared around these here parts. You started something. Finish it.
80. Sam: Mom--uh--she belches.
81. Dr.: She belches.
82. Sam: Consistently, repeatedly, and disgustingly.
83. Mrs. B.: That's right. I swallow air. I went to a doctor many years ago about it. It's a nervous habit, and when I'm very upset, evidently I swallow--
84. Sam: Why were you so upset tonight?
85. Mrs. B.: Tonight was not for that, Sam.
86. Dr.: Sam, when Mama belches, whom does she, whose face does she belch into?
87. Mr. B.: Mine mostly.
88. Sam: His! (laughing and pointing vigorously to father)
89. Dr.: His. (all laugh)
90. Mr. B.: Mine, if you like, or anybody else who happens around.
91. Sam: Only with her choice friends she refrains (sic) herself. Somehow she doesn't swallow air when her good friends are around, her high class friends (sarcastically).
92. Mrs. B.: That's right. It's not high class, Sam.

93. Sam: Yes, it is.
94. Mrs. B.: No, I wouldn't call it high class.
95. Sam: But you manage not to swallow air--
96. Mrs. B.: Well, let me read what's in here (picks up notebook). Maybe this will give you a better idea--
97. Dr.: Well, one moment now. Is that the only--
98. Sam: That's about the worst habit she has.
99. Dr.: --habit, in your eyes?
100. Sam: Yeah, that's about the worst of it.
101. Dr.: That's the worst? No others?
102. Sam: (giggles) No, I haven't got the nerve.
103. Dr.: Come on, come on.
104. Sam: No, no, really. that's about all.
105. Mrs. B.: Now I don't know what else he has reference to.
106. Dr.: You know you're only playing a game now. That isn't fair.
107. Sam: I'm sorry. I'm not going to say anything else.
108. Dr.: Now he's tensing up because he knows all about Mama's habits.
109. Sam: Then ask him (points to father, laughing embarrassedly).
110. Dr.: No, I want to ask you first. You started this.
111. Sam: I'm sorry. I'm not going to tell you.
112. Dr.: (perceiving Ann smiling broadly) Ann, Ann's got a trick up her sleeve, too.
113. Sam: I can't tell you that, Dr.
114. Dr.: Oh, come on.
115. Sam: I'm sorry, I can't.
116. Mr. B.: He doesn't want to embarrass his mother.
117. Mrs. B.: I don't know what he has reference to so I don't--
118. Dr.: You're a teaser, Sam--
119. Sam: I'm sorry, I--
120. Dr.: --a teaser.
121. Sam: I can't.
122. Dr.: You start to begin to commence to say something about your Ma. You make a big promise and all of a sudden you fade out. That's not cricket.
123. Sam: No, well, that's about the worst thing.

124. Dr.: I know your Ma is impatient. She's looking at her--
125. Mrs. B.: No, I was just--
126. Dr.: --at her record.
127. Mrs. B.: No, that's not impatience. I was just--looking at it (the notebook). But he's not saying anything so I've nothing to listen to.
128. Sam: No, I'll tell you the truth. I really don't have anything--I'm not going to say.
129. Mr. B.: Might as well ask somebody else.
130. Dr.: If you don't say, it's going to come out in the wash anyway.
131. Sam: So let it come out.
132. Dr.: It might as well come out where it started.
133. Sam: I'm sorry. I will not do it (emphatically)!
134. Dr.: (again noticing Ann) Ann, do you want to speak up ahead of Pop?
135. Mr. B.: Come on, Ann.
136. (Ann hides head in her arms. Sam puts his arm around Ann in a friendly way and whispers to her.)
137. Mrs. B.: Oh, look now, you're wasting--
138. Sam: Come on, Ann.
139. Ann: I'm finished. Mommy's a nut. Daddy's a nut.
140. Sam: I'll say they are!
141. Dr.: Always belching in Pop's face.
142. (Mrs. B. and Ann laugh.)
143. Dr.: Oh, Mom likes that! Look at her giggle!
144. Mrs. B.: You know why I'm giggling?
145. Dr.: Why?
146. Mrs. B.: I asked Jack as a favor to me, when I realized that I was going to do this, that he should keep some kind of a record of our relationship. I feel there's lots to be desired in it. Maybe if we can get it down on paper, you can help us with it. So--he--did do it for several days. Last night, I said, "Please write that thing for me. Because I want to know." I knew I had written it down. So he did write it down. And there were several things he wrote that were mostly about things that I don't care to discuss in front of the children. However, one of the things was about the belching. And I giggled because I

refuse to take it seriously. I know it's nothing terrible. It's, it's a nervousness. And so I, I giggle. Now as a result of that giggling, evidently, it put him in a different frame of mind. And after he said he would not let me see his paper until after I let him read what I had written. Well, some of this stuff is pretty--rugged. I mean, it's, it's what I think and it's not complimentary in some respects. But he read it and for the first time since we're married, which is twenty years, he *didn't* get--

147. Mr. B.: More, dear.

148. Mrs. B.: All right, it's a little more than twenty. He didn't get angry. And I can honestly say that's the first time that he ever acted like the kind of man I hoped he was. (Father sighs deeply.) He didn't get angry with, with it--at this notebook. Well, of course he didn't--

149. Dr.: Oh, my, my. That's quite a bit of progress. Last week, you said he wasn't no man at all.

150. Mrs. B.: Most of the time he, he does not react the way I would like him to. I can honestly say this is the first time he acted the way I would like him to and the way I would expect him to, the first time since we're married. It was a pleasure to see him *not* get angry at something that was the truth, and he, and it was, there was a sense of humor in it, and it just lovely. And I, I would appreciate so much--

151. Dr.: You mean Jack has a temper with you?

152. Mrs. B.: Yes; he's either too good or too bad.

153. Dr.: Too good or too bad. (Notices Jack protruding his tongue) Look at his tongue.

154. Mrs. B.: He can be a son of a bee or he can be an angel. And he doesn't always follow the middle course. Either he's too easy to get along with or for nothing he'll--

155. Dr.: I asked you to look at his tongue.

156. Mrs. B.: Well, I didn't see his tongue.

157. Dr.: Why don't you look?

158. Mrs. B.: Well, I was talking to you so I was looking at you.

159. Dr.: Why do you have eyes for me only? What about Jack?
160. Mrs. B.: Well, I think that when you talk to somebody, you should look at him, which is something he doesn't do. Which I have criticized--
161. Mr. B.: (noting Mrs. B.'s pointing finger) Did you see that finger go? (laughs loudly)
162. Mrs. B.: Which is something I have criticized him for many times. I think--
163. Dr.: Well, what did you want to talk about that he had his tongue in a very special position?
164. Ann: (gestures) Like this.
165. Mrs. B.: Well, I don't know why. I don't know why at all. He was laughing to himself. I don't know why.
166. Dr.: (to Jack) Did you see what happened?
167. Mr. B.: No, no. I would really appreciate it if you'd tell me.
168. Dr.: (to Ann) How do you feel about that tongue of his?
169. Ann: I thought it was funny.
170. Dr.: (to Jack) What were you about to do with your tongue?
171. Sam: What a family!
172. Mr. B.: It happens that my putting my tongue out is a habit (all laugh). It's a habit of maybe forty or forty-five years. Whenever I write, I can just sign my name, my tongue will be out.
173. Dr.: You mean you stick your tongue out whenever you concentrate?
174. Mr. B.: Whenever I do anything--
175. Ann: I know something I could say, but Sam would kill me and so would my father, so I can't.
176. Mrs. B.: Nobody is going to kill you, Ann.
177. Mr. B.: Nobody will kill you.
178. Ann: Sam will, Sam will.
179. Mrs. B.: Sam won't kill you either. Nobody kills around here.
180. Dr.: All right, spit it out, Ann. Let's hear.
181. Mrs. B.: Come on, Ann.
182. Ann: Sam, Sam--
183. Dr.: What were you going to say?
184. Mrs. B.: Go ahead.

185. (Sam turns completely away from group, so that his back is turned to the camera and to the group members. He maintains this position for most of the remainder of this session, until the interaction noted in items 334 through 340.)

186. Ann: Today, he had a date with a girl and he locked the door, and when I was at the door, he said, "You're going to be in so much trouble!" And I think he likes the girl more than he does me, because whenever I have a date, he, I never lock the door. When I, I had to get something in the kitchen--and he, and it was locked when I--knocked. And he said, "I have to tell her that I don't like her." And then I found out that he was lying about that. And I don't think it's right to lock the door--because--Renee and Helen, we had to go around the back way and he wouldn't let us in.

187. Dr.: Shows what your brother, Sam, did to you.

188. Mrs. B.: That's another thing about Sam. He, he's like his father in that respect. He's either too good or too bad. Either he's an angel and, and a doll; or, for no reason at all, he'll blow his top and simply not be fit to live with.

189. Dr.: (notices Ann grinning, making faces, and bidding for attention) See, as you were concentrating, you didn't see what Ann was doing with her top.

190. Ann: (giggles)

191. Mrs. B.: Now, I hope Sam isn't angry after this session.

192. Mr. B.: I was going to say that in my opinion, this is the case with most people, although Joan seems to think that this is a problem that we have a corner of the market on. I think that most people tend to go to either of two extremes. I think it's the unusual person who steers a steady, middle-of-the-road course constantly. I haven't yet met that person.

193. Mrs. B.: Well, I think that's true, "constantly." But to get unduly upset over nothing, and, and raise the roof, and get really nasty and mean--
194. Dr.: How does he do that?
195. Mrs. B.: Well, if I read these notes, you'll know how he does it. Otherwise, I can't really describe it to you, my inner feelings. That's the only way--
196. Dr.: Before you read your notes now, I'd just like to ask Jack one question. When you belch in Jack's face--
197. Mrs. B.: (interrupting) Well, I don't deliberately do that.
198. Dr.: Excuse me.
199. Mrs. B.: I don't deliberately do that.
200. Dr.: How does, how does it feel?
201. Mr. B.: Well, her belching does something to me that, that I just can't explain, with as good a command of English that I think I do have. It is just like waving a red flag in front of my face. And has for years to the point where we went to doctors in Woodmere and with no satisfaction.
202. Ann: (interrupting) Sam--
203. Mr. B.: And the thing that aggravates me more than anything is that with certain company, although she pleads that this is uncontrollable, and that she has no control over it, with certain company in the house, she can control it beautifully.
204. Dr.: Well now, when was the last time she belched in your face?
205. Mr. B.: Last night.
206. Mrs. B.: No, no, no.
207. Mr. B.: Please don't say "no," because you belched--
208. Mrs. B.: (interrupting) Most of the time--
209. Mr. B.: --when I--The minute she gets into bed, she starts belching like mad.
210. Dr.: In bed?
211. Mr. B.: Yes.
212. Mrs. B.: Yes, I think it's psychological.
213. Mr. B.: Yes, the minute she gets into bed. Yes.

214. Mrs. B.: I really think there is something psychological. I'm not feeling now. When I lie down, I begin to swallow air. I don't know why. And there are some times I don't do it, but on the whole, when I--

215. (Sam turns to Ann while his mother is talking. He smiles with Ann, puts his arm around her, whispers something, and then again turns away from group.)

216. Ann: (interrupting) Excuse me, but just now he--

217. Mrs. B.: All right (trying to resume).

218. Ann: He said, "If you tell about that lipstick mark, I'll kill you!"

219. Mr. B.: Oh, stop it now!

220. Mrs. B.: Sam, you're being as silly as, as I would expect you to be now.

221. Ann: I'm going to bring it out.

222. Dr.: As soon as I begin concentrating on the love life between Ma and Pa, you two kids start cutting up.

223. Sam: I'm sorry, but I don't like it one bit. (still turned away from group)

224. Ann: (raises hand) He--

225. Dr.: (to Sam) Would you rather talk about your love life?

226. Sam: No. I'd rather talk about nobody's love life.

227. Ann: I'd like to say something.

228. Dr.: Yes, Ann.

229. Ann: Well, he has a mark on his neck. And I was teasing him and saying it was lipstick from his girlfriend. And he said, "If you say that in front of Dr. A., I'll murder you." And I didn't like that--what he said.

230. Mrs. B.: Sam has not got a sense of humor when it comes to things he's touchy about. He doesn't want to discuss his report card, which I said I would discuss tonight. And he said, "You'd better not, or else." And I think it's a very important things to discuss.

231. Dr.: Sam--

232. Mrs. B.: (interrupting) Would you mind turning around and acting like a man?

233. Mr. B.: Sam.
234. Dr.: He's angry. It's--
235. Mrs. B.: (interrupting) I can see he's angry at me, too, now.
236. (Ann whispers with her mother and changes places with her.)
237. Mrs. B.: Now, please turn around. (Sam continues facing away.)
238. Dr.: Now, we were--
239. Mrs. B.: Yes.
240. Dr.: --talking about his special date with his girlfriend and Ann felt so alone. Because, after all, Sam's your boyfriend, isn't he?
241. Ann: No.
242. Dr.: No?
243. Ann: No. Never had one.
244. Dr.: Is it bad? But Sam is also sore at me because he doesn't like it when--
245. Ann: (interrupting) He doesn't like it because--
246. Dr.: --when we talk about, talk to Ma and Pa here about their love life. He doesn't like that at all. He wants to pretend like he knows nothing at all about their love life.
247. (Mother puts arm on Sam's shoulder and tries to turn him back to group.)
248. Mrs. B.: Will you--?
249. Sam: Stop touching me!
250. Mrs. B.: Well, will you turn around and act like--
251. Sam: I don't feel like it.
252. Mrs. B.: I know you don't feel like it, but turn around anyway.
253. Sam: (makes barely audible, objecting sound)
254. Dr.: Sam, you're angry at me, not Ma.
255. Sam: No, I'm not angry at you. I'm angry at my sister and my mother.
256. Ann: Just because I told the truth.
257. Sam: Why don't you learn to shut up for a change?
258. Ann: Why don't you shut up?
259. Dr.: Ann, when you changed seats, you wanted to get away from your brother. Are you angry at him?
260. Ann: Yes.
261. Mrs. B.: You see--
262. Dr.: (interrupting) You didn't like it when he had that girl in the apartment?
263. Ann: No.

264. Dr.: What were you so sore about?

265. Ann: Because I had nothing to do. And I wanted to get something out of the kitchen, and he told me to go out.

266. Dr.: Well, he wanted a little privacy with his girlfriend.

267. Ann: In a smooch.

268. Dr.: Smooch. Well, what's wrong with a smooch?

269. Mr. B.: What's wrong with that?

270. Ann: Because he had marks on his neck.

271. Sam: Will you shut up!

272. Mrs. B.: Sam, you're acting so babyish.

273. Sam: Will you, will you, please, too.

274. Dr.: Don't you think a guy like Sam can smooch a little bit with a girl, and get some lipstick on his neck.

275. Ann: (whispers) It's wrong.

276. Dr.: What? It's wrong? It's bad?

277. Ann: (whisper) Yes.

278. Dr.: The only thing I know that's bad about it is that he got the lipstick on his neck.

279. Ann: Yeah, so it's evidence.

280. Dr.: Oh, you want to hang the man on evidence.

281. Ann: When we leave, he's going to murder me.

282. Dr.: You're not going to smooch?

283. Ann: No.

284. Dr.: What are you going to do?

285. Ann: Nothing.

286. Mrs. B.: What was that game you were playing at your dance, with a bottle in the middle of the room spinning around? Huh?

287. Dr.: Anyhow, anyhow you two kids just--

288. Ann: I didn't get lipstick.

289. Dr.: You two kids just pulled us right out of your parents' bed. We were in there in the double bed. Mom was belching in Pop's face and that's where you interrupted the story. Now, Joan, you say it's psychological.

290. Mrs. B.: I felt--

291. Dr.: The moment you go to bed with Jack--

292. Mrs. B.: Not the moment. I wouldn't put it quite so--uh, like that. But I do--uh--begin to swallow air and I don't know why. I really don't. Now, maybe what I have written here will have some bearing on the subject.

293. Dr.: Well, you can read that in just a moment. Seems you hurt Jack's feeling, torment him no end. He can't stand it when you belch in his face. Is that right?

294. Mr. B.: Did you ever try, or think that you wanted to kiss a woman, and just when you're about to do it, have her belch in your face?

295. Ann: (giggles loudly)

296. Dr.: I'm terribly sympathetic with you.

297. Ann: (giggles again)

298. Mr. B.: I mean--

299. Dr.: It's really not what I would call kissing.

300. Mr. B.: I mean--this is something!--Unless you wear a gas mask!

301. (Mrs. B. and Ann giggle together almost uncontrollably.)

302. Dr.: Smells bad?

303. Mr. B.: Blows your head to one side and it's really very unhealthy. And I just hope you never have, have the--

304. Dr.: Exposure to gas?

305. (Mrs. B. and Ann continue to giggle, even louder now.)

306. Mr. B.: Yes, specifically.

307. Dr.: At the moment you wanted to kiss her.

308. Mr. B.: Well, you're afraid. I'm serious. I--

309. Mrs. B.: Well, I think this is just part of an excuse on his part, really. Because I don't do it that often, or every night.

310. Ann: Just now!

311. Mr. B.: You do it that often and you do it--

213. Mrs. B.: Believe me when I tell you I don't. I, I cannot--it does not happen every night or anything like that. There are nights--

313. Mr. B.: I didn't say it happened every night.

314. Mrs. B.: All right.

315. Mr. B.: There are nights when you will blame it on what you've eaten. There will be nights when you'll blame it on what you've drank. There'll be nights when you'll blame it on being upset. And other nights, you'll blame it on not sleeping enough the day before. (Joan and Ann are giggling.) And you will not always have an excuse, but the belching is there.

316. Dr.: Ann, she just loves this. (Ann giggles.) Oh, boy, does she love it!

317. Mr. B.: I'm not saying it was done deliberately, but--

318. Dr.: (to Ann) You raised your hand. What did you want to say?

319. Ann: I want you to see the marks on Sam's neck.

320. Sam: Oh, never mind!

321. Ann: You want to stop it, I know. But I want to get him as mad as he got me today.

322. Dr.: Now, just a minute. We're in your parents' bed. Can we stay there a few minutes? Or won't you let us? (brief silence) Now, (to Ann) suppose you move over again next to Sam, because we've got a problem between Ma and Pa here. We got to know what to do with this gas.

323. Ann: I don't want to go near him. (But she moves back, next to Sam.)

324. Mrs. B.: Well, I'll leave out anything that has to do with bed. Because if it's going to disturb them, then I think it should be left out.

325. Sam: (angrily) It disturbs me.

326. Dr.: I notice--

327. Sam: It's disturbed me for the last ten minutes.

328. Dr.: I know that. You're mad at me. Because last week you said you didn't want to be here and we had to stop. Would you rather leave the room? (no answer) Sam?

329. Sam: I wouldn't like to answer that.

330. Dr.: It isn't really that you don't know about this stuff. You just want to make out you don't know about this stuff.

331. (Mrs. B. whispers to Ann.)

332. Sam: (still turned aside from group) I don't want you to talk about it in my presence. I'm willing to talk about anything you want, which I think is wrong, if anyone else is present, but I don't want to be present.

333. Mrs. B.: Well, why don't you leave?

334. Sam: All right, I'll leave. (Gets up and moves toward door.)

335. Mrs. B.: It's perfectly all right. You can wait outside.

336. (All talk at once. Dr. restrains Sam as he is leaving.)

337. Mr. B.: Wait a minute. Wait a minute. Let Dr. A. decide whether Sam is to leave or not.
338. Mrs. B.: Well, I'm sorry. I thought--
339. Dr.: Okay. Sit down.
340. (Sam then takes his chair and now faces group.)
341. Dr.: If we come to a point, Sam, where it seems really sensible for both children to leave, I'll ask both of you to leave. If we want to deal with the <u>very</u> private part in the relations between Ma and Pa. But I want to know what bothers you so much.
342. Sam: It bothers me.
343. Dr.: I know it bothers you.
344. Sam: I don't know why; it just bothers me.
345. Ann: I don't want to go out of here even at the private part because, because he's going to kill me if I go out.
346. Dr.: (to Sam) Why so much?
347. Sam: I don't know; it just bothers me.
348. Dr.: Yeah, but it would be very interesting to, to try to understand--
349. Sam: I really, I really wouldn't mind--
350. Dr.: --why you act so terribly--
351. Sam: Well, I don't know. It just, it just bothers me.
352. Dr.: You know that every Ma and Pa kiss.
353. Sam: I certainly do, but that--
354. Dr.: So what's the trouble?
355. Sam: It bothers me. I don't know what the trouble is. It bothers me.
356. Dr.: Do you think, since we're all here together--
357. Sam: No, I'll tell you why it bothers me, if you want to know--
358. Dr.: --that you make an attempt with us and see--
359. Sam: No, I'll tell you exactly why it bothers me. Because just like it bothers me that Ann is citing my private business, which I entrusted to her to just mind her own business. I didn't even ask her to, to bother me, when she, she insisted on bothering me. I told her something about, you know I wanted to tell the girl that I didn't like her, so she should please leave me alone. But what I do is my business and I think that what my parents do is their business. I may be very wrong. I--maybe it's everyone else's busi-

ness. But I don't like it and I, I would rather not, be present if you, or whoever wants it, wants to discuss it.

360. Dr.: Now, Sam--

361. Ann: Just now--

362. Dr.: --you don't want to be in on a thing that we talked about, the private love life between Ma and Pa, because if you are, you're afraid that Ma and Pa, and I, too, might invade your private love life.

363. Sam: No, that, that isn't possible, because I do not feel that way. Because *nobody* knows about my private love life except me. And--

364. Ann: And me.

365. Sam: --and that's the way it's going to stay as far as I'm concerned.

366. Dr.: You insist on your privacy.

367. Sam: That's right.

368. Dr.: Well, all right. Look, I can't keep you here. The door is wide open, but I would prefer, if you can tolerate it, that you stay with us, because I'm interested in helping the whole family. Even if it bothers you--

369. Sam: As long as you don't let Ann know, that's all I care about. As long as you know it annoys me.

370. Dr.: --just to hear something.

371. Sam: Well, all right. Whatever you say, Dr.

372. Dr.: Now, that's very good. Now, you let me know if it's too much for you because--

373. Sam: Well, as far as I'm concerned, the second it began was too much for me, because I don't like it. But if, as far as if you want me to stay--

374. Dr.: I'd prefer it.

375. Sam: Okay. Whatever you say.

376. Dr.: Good. (Ann raises her hand.) Ann.

377. Ann: Well, I, I don't want to go home tonight because he's gonna--

378. Sam: (in great exasperation) I, I--did I ever hit you or harm you?

379. Ann: Oh, today.

380. Sam: Well, I never did. So just be quiet.

381. Dr.: Well, do you think he ought to kill you because of what you did, talking about his smooching?

382. Ann: Well, I--
383. Dr.: Do you think he ought to kill you?
384. Ann: Well, I saw those marks on his neck all right. Look if they're not lipstick.
385. Dr.: Well, I already saw them. So what? What's terrible about that?
386. Ann: And telling me that story that he doesn't do anything. And--and--and he--and Sam was so mean to me. He, he, he, he was mad at me. He wanted me to call up my friend when he heard that she was coming, so that we wouldn't peek in on him, and so that he would have privacy with his girlfriend. And, and--
387. Dr.: Well, now, don't you think when, when you're Sam's age, you'll want a little bit of privacy with your boyfriend?
388. Ann: Yeah, but if, if I had a little brother that had a date, and I wouldn't tell him to break the date.
389. Mr. B.: Because he can't be sure you wouldn't invade his privacy. That's why.
390. Dr.: Well, we'll, we'll settle this later, but he didn't do anything terrible.
391. Ann: And he locked the door. And when I knocked he, he came out stamping his feet and yelling at me.
392. Dr.: I think you're just jealous of that girl he had in there. That's all.
393. (Sam laughs)
394. Ann: I'm not jealous of that ugly girl.
395. Dr.: Oh! She was ugly, was she?
396. Ann: Yes.
397. Dr.: You mean you're better looking?
398. Sam: I'm going to smack her right in the face if she doesn't shut her mouth. Look (to father), do you mind if I leave?
399. Mr. B.: No, I don't mind.
400. Sam: (gets up and starts to leave)
401. Dr.: Wait a minute. (Sam leaves room.)
402. Mrs. B.: You see, what Sam is doing now is what he does at home, which I think is inexcusable. I feel that this child should have a great deal more control over himself than he has.

403. Dr.: Well, you're a good preacher. I agree he ought to, but he doesn't. There are--

404. Mrs. B.: That's right.

405. Dr.: --reasons for that--

406. Mrs. B.: I'm disturbed about what he just did.

407. Dr.: --It's about Ann. (to Ann) You say his girl was ugly. Are you much prettier than she?

408. Ann: I think so.

409. Dr.: Oh, you're pretty jealous of her.

410. Ann: I am *not* jealous of her.

411. Dr.: Oh, you're teasing now.

412. Ann: I'm not.

413. Dr.: You're a pretty good romancer yourself. Like to tease a lot, you and Sam both. Well, anyhow, let's be back to Ma and Pa. Is that all right with you, Ann? Hm? Well now, what did you do last night when she belched in your face? You wanted to kiss her and she belched.

414. Mr. B.: No, I didn't want to kiss her. I merely said that that is my reaction. You asked what my reaction is and why I resent it, or why it upsets me, and I merely said it is very unhappy to kiss a woman and have her belch in your face.

415. Dr.: Hmm.

416. Mr. B.: Now, that doesn't mean that every time I attempt to kiss my wife she does it. But--it can happen more often than not.

417. Dr.: Well, you know, you, you sound so reasonable right now that I don't believe a word that's coming out of your mouth. You're not that reasonable when you get belched at. Are you?

418. Mr. B.: Well, it annoys me to the point where I have--

419. Dr.: It does.

420. Mr. B.: Yes. I have turned around and I have at times left the bed and gone inside and read the newspaper, and read a magazine or done other things. I've criticized her for it.

421. Ann: Can I please go out now?

422. Dr.: Well we're going to bring Sam back in here in a little bit.

423. Ann: I'll come back if he starts to hit me.

424. Dr.: You want to be with him?
425. Ann: No, I want to go out. (leaves room)
426. Dr.: All right, folks, here's your chance to talk plain English.
(From here the session continues without either of the children present.)

The Interaction of Verbal and Non-verbal Behavior and Its Therapeutic Significance

Within the context of our script there are certain relationships between verbal and non-verbal expressions which are evident. Perhaps the most obvious relationship is that of the inverse relationship between overt speech and non-verbal expression.

The verbal productivity of the group members is given in Table I. Three separate indices are used. The total number of words used gives a general indication of total verbal output. The number of items may indicate the proneness to intervene verbally or to respond to the therapeutic intervention. The number of items with twenty-five or more words may reveal the member's ability to hold the floor, so to speak, and the number of words in these twenty-five or more word items could indicate the member's tenacity in floor-holding.

Table I

Verbal Productivity of Group Members

	Total Number of Words	Total Number of Items	No. of Items with 25 or More Words	No. of Words in 25+ Words
Dr. A.	1593	153	13	511
Mr. B.	679	52	7	370
Mrs. B.	1480	78	17	933
Sam	720	79	4	229
Ann	559	58	3	234

Table I demonstrates that Mrs. B. is more productive verbally than any other family member. Dr. A. does produce more words and also more items. He productivity, however, consists to a large extent of brief therapeutic interventions. Mrs. B. is the most determined "floorholder" and produces the largest quantity of words in this capacity. These data do thus support the inverse relationship posited between verbal productivity and non-verbal expressiveness. Mrs. B., who makes the fewest gestures (see below), does most of the talking. Since we are mainly concerned with the specific non-verbal expressions in their clinical context, the data of Table I will not be analyzed in more detail.

Let us focus now upon the interaction between verbal and non-verbal behavior for each individual in the family, especially as this is responded to by the therapist. Look, for example, at Item 28, where Dr. A. reacts to the father's gesture rather than to Sam's remarks of the moment. Mr. B. responds to Dr. A.'s interpretation with a loud laugh, which in itself contains both release and defiance.

At Item 51 Mr. B. picks at his finger and the therapist immediately uses this gesture to open up an entire channel of inquiry. The whole subject of "disgusting habits" stems from this single observation, although the object of attention shifts from Mr. B. to Mrs. B. Mr. B. seems quite expert at averting inquiry, while Mrs. B. apparently takes on a scapegoat role (2) most readily at this point. Mrs. B.'s belching, another non-verbal expression, becomes the fulcrum about which the remainder of the session revolves.

Sam's attitude of provocative reticence is the channel through which the therapist is able to approach the parents' sexual conflict. It is of interest to note that the subject of belching and sex is again opened by a gesture interpretation (see Item 79). Sam exhibits two basic behavioral gestures in this session. The first is that of pointing vigorously to his father (Items 88 and 109). This gesture has both accusation and warmth, a kind of laughingly pointing to the perpetrator of the deed. It is as if Sam wants to turn the spotlight on the masked hero (or villain) and induce him to remove his disguise.

Sam's second gesture is that of turning entirely away from the group. He actually spends the major part of this session with his back turned to his family (Items 185 to 340) and soon after he does turn back to the group, Sam gets up and leaves the room. It is clear that Sam wants to remove his name entirely from the cast of players. And yet there is a kind of pretense to Sam's withdrawal. Despite his apparent wish to leave, he both attracts attention and provokes anger by turning his back. Sam's very efforts to flee make him conspicuous and a topic of family concern.

In addition, Sam's apparent withdrawal has a hidden face. Although his verbal expressions to his sister are angry accusation, his behavioral gestures are warm and affectionate. He smiles warmly at Ann and puts his arm around her in a friendly fashion (Item 215). This behavior is quite contradictory to overt verbalization and would probably not be detected without motion picture recording.

Mr. B. has a number of small gestures. He sighs (Item 1), beckons with his hand (Item 28), picks at his finger (Item 51) and sticks out his tongue (Item 153). None of these escape the attention of his therapist. It is as if Mr. B. is trying to remain unnoticed, but is betrayed by involuntary cues, which demonstrate his instigatory role in the family circle.

Ann's gestures are not yet so definitely developed. She demonstrates with her whole body and by facial grimaces. Ann makes faces (Item 112), raises her hand (Item 134), hides her head (Item 136) or merely interrupts (Item 175). She cannot fully express herself in words and must take her part by actions and facial masks; this is primitive drama.

It is of interest that Mrs. B., who during this session reveals almost no behavioral gestures but sits rather stiffly and with frozen facial expression, speaks far more than any other family member. It is as if words take the place of actions that cannot come forth. Nevertheless, such suppressed activity has come out in the secret family life. Mrs. B. belches and is unable to control this involuntary betrayal of hostility. When the subject of belching is discussed, Mrs. B. and Ann go into uncontrollable giggles (Items 301, 305 and 315), which may demonstrate a conspiratorial alliance between the women of the family. In one sense Mrs. B.'s frozen face is itself a form of nonverbal expression, as is the entire gamut of facial expressions and mannerisms. Mrs. B. is the only family member who does not laugh on her own, and she communicates a sense of emotional isolation which may be related to her lack of non-verbal expressiveness.

There are numerous interpretations that can be made of the individual gestures and in fact the major therapeutic movement in this session arises from Dr. A.'s reflecting of gestures (Items 28 and 79) and calling attention to them. Thus Sam's frequent laughing may be a clue to his repressed aggression and inability to assert himself. Mr. B.'s sighs and movements with his tongue reveal his frustrated oral cravings.

Perhaps the most significant behavioral gestures are those of Sam putting his arm around Ann in a friendly way and whispering to her. His affectionate attitude in this behavior is quite at odds with the overt verbal communication, since the friendliness between the siblings is contradicted by their bitter quarreling. By analyzing the total behavioral sequence one can see that Sam provokes his sister into instigating his own aggression. He seems to provoke Ann's first contribution to the session (Items 136, 139: "Mommy's a nut; Daddy's a nut!") and then feels free to corroborate her comment (Item 140).

Later (Item 215) he smiles broadly at Ann, while threatening to kill her if she gives away his secret. Of course Ann complies with Sam's wish to interrupt the proceedings and, as Dr. A. notes, the children succeed in steering the conversation away from the topic of parental sex.

The most significant non-verbal behavior is that occurring outside this session: (1) Mrs. B.'s belching, (2) Mrs. B.'s notebook, and (3) Sam's lipstick mark. Therapeutic progress has already brought all of this behavior into treatment process.

Non-verbal Cues and the Re-enactment of Conflict

Let us turn from interpretations of gestures and behavior to some structural relationships within these data. It is our impression that the verbal communications among family members are cued by certain key gestures. On a relatively overt level we have seen how Sam cued Ann to interrupt an unwelcome topic of conversation. However, what about the gesture where Mrs. B. puts her hand on Sam's shoulder to persuade him to turn back to the family circle (Item 247)? This gesture, as seen on the film, seems more studied and artificial than spontaneous. Sam's immediate reaction is one of intense annoyance, but his only expression is a grunt. Dr. A. tries to clarify Sam's anger but then Ann again lends herself as a target of displaced hostility. In this sequence we can perceive (1) inadequate mothering, (2) reactive anger from Sam, and (3) Ann's provocative drawing of the anger from Mrs. B. to herself. The sequence thus illustrates the crucial traumatic interaction of this family in encapsulated miniature.

Let us examine Mr. B.'s tongue gesture (Item 153) and the behavior in which it is embedded. Mrs. B. and the therapist are engaged in an analysis of her husband's behavior, and she is expressing her pleasure at "the first time he ever acted like the kind of man I hoped he was." Mr. B. sighed deeply at this comment, and Mrs. B. went on to say that her pleasure arose mainly from her husband's lack of anger at reading what she had written about him. Dr. A. interprets Mr. B.'s manhood and his temper, and then the tongue emerged.

It is clear that Mrs. B.'s concept of masculinity is a significantly inverted one. Acceptable masculinity to her means compliance to her own wishes and a lack of aggression, but in twenty years of marriage she has been unable to get Mr. B. to accede completely to the passive role she would like to assign. Now Mrs. B. feels that therapy has succeeded in getting her husband to see the light. This was "the first time that he ever acted like the kind of man I hoped he was. He didn't get angry . . . ."

Mr. B.'s tongue gesture is soon mimicked by Ann, who also sticks her tongue out. When Dr. A. tries to clarify this interaction, Ann again evades him. She says merely that she thought her father was being funny, and then changes the subject back to Sam (Item 175). It is at this point that Sam turns his back on the family group.

Here we see a series of role inductions that starts with a conflict of role definition (masculine assertiveness) expressed by the mother, is transmuted into a gestural displacement by the father, which in turn is mimicked and side-tracked by the daughter, which then leads to the withdrawal from the family by the son. Again we have the total family conflict triggered and illustrated in miniature by a brief family exchange of non-verbal gestures.

Mr. B. is unable to take the appropriate role of assertive paternal responsibility. His wife expresses her dissatisfaction in terms of the fact that "he does not react the way I would like him to." Mr. B.'s inner conflict is unverbalized, but comes out in a gesture of his tongue. Ann mimics and makes fun of her father's plight, and then turns the spotlight on her brother. She verbalizes her father's latent rage and expresses it in terms of "Sam would kill me me and so would my father." Sam is immediately provoked to leave the scene. This sequence may well reproduce the conflict that originally brought the family to treatment. That is, the daughter embodies the unexpressed but violent antagonisms of her parents. When she confronts her brother with this violence, he suddenly fades out of the scene. Does this not recall the incident in which Ann threatened Sam with a knife and he then fell in a dead faint in the parents' bedroom?

We could use these instances of miniature re-living of the family conflict as a way of conceptualizing one mode of effectiveness of family therapy. That is, family treatment offers the opportunity to mitigate the traumatic effects of conflict by re-inducing them in therapy and gaining insight into their origins and effects. In this process there is no doubt that the role of the family therapist is paramount and we turn now to an analysis of the therapist-family interactions.

It is clear that Dr. A. is the most active member of the group. He is continually trying to impart meaning to the behavior that takes place and he confronts each family member with the implications of the material that emerges. In addition, there is therapeutic effort to improve communication among the family and to permit each member to express opinions and feelings that have lain dormant. The subject of belching is a good example of behavior that has emerged for examination and discussion as a result of Dr. A.'s direct prompting and encouragement.

It is significant to note that Dr. A. is interested both in specific material that is being withheld and also in improving the over-all efficiency of family communication. These two factors are interrelated, and it is a therapeutic challenge to attend simultaneously to both of them. The way in which this task is accomplished is well illustrated quite early in the session, at Item 28. Dr. A. had been prompting and encouraging Sam to express his feelings about his father. However, at the moment that Sam seems ready to reveal some material, the therapist interrupts to call attention to a gesture on Mr. B.'s part and he compares this to Mrs. B.'s gesture. This therapeutic maneuver brings Mrs. B. into the session for the first time. She brings up the "anecdotal record" that she has been keeping, and this is the material that later in the session leads to her comments about the "kind of man" she wants her husband to be. Thus, by attending to both non-verbal cues and reluctance to be direct in expression, the therapist is able to uncover the subtle structure of family communication.

If we put all of this material together, we can see a unity to the family therapy session that emerges. There are various cues, verbal and non-verbal, that prompt each family member to re-enact the traumas and conflicts that led the family to seek treatment. We see the family drama re-lived in miniature scenes, each of which reproduces the family conflict and the member's place in it. The therapist may then be seen as a kind of director or stage manager, who sets the scene and elicits the dialogue and stage action.

The factor that seems to lend most unity to the session is the total family interaction, which seems to have a quality of dramatic destiny. It is as though each family member is taking a role determined by an underlying plot design that has its own independence and intention. Thus, Mrs. B. comes into marriage and must then participate in a husband-wife team. She wants her husband to "act like a man," but her concept of this role has been conditioned by her father, who "was a horror." Soon there is a son, who also seems to Mrs. B. to be "a horror," and later there is a daughter, who does not take the role her mother assigns to her and thus becomes a discipline problem.

Mr. B., who came from a divorced home, was raised to be "independent." Now, as a father, he tends to remain aloof from the battle. He assigns the role of disciplinarian to his wife, but at the same time mocks her (Item 161) in order to call attention away from his own role inadequacy (Item 153) and to undercut her authority, which he senses should belong to him.

Sam and Ann reproduce the provocative inconsistencies of their mother and father. Thus Sam incites Ann to antagonize him, and he in turn withdraws from the family in the same way his father abdicates his role. Ann similarly follows her mother in making fun of the masculine image of aggression ("Sam's going to kill me.") but at the same time is overcome by her own aggressive impulses that she cannot control.

Non-verbal cues during this family session also illustrate a kind of hypocrisy on the part of the parents. Mr. and Mrs. B. have, on the surface of things, demanded certain forms of behavior from their children. Thus Mrs. B. asks Sam to act "like a man" and rejoin the family circle (Item 232), but her act of touching him has the actual effect of reinforcing his apparent rejection of the family (Items 247-253). Sam is quite "touchy" (Item 230) in his relationship with his mother, and here it is clear that her non-verbal behavior plays a direct role in instigating his touchiness. Mrs. B.'s words ask for one form of behavior but her actions elicit another. In some respects this contradiction resembles the "double-bind" situation, as described by Bateson and others (3, 12).

Mr. B., on the other hand, often makes perfunctory efforts to appear as the authority and disciplinarian of the family. Thus he insists that Sam respond to Dr. A.'s question (Item 26). However, at the same time that he makes this presumably authoritative demand, he simultaneously makes a hand gesture (Item 26) which betrays his own need to be given to rather than to direct the actions of others. When this need of Mr. B. is interpreted by the therapist (Item 28), Mr. B. laughs his acknowledgement and Sam merely continues his provocative withholding.

There is thus a power vacuum in this family, attributable to a mother with a distorted concept of masculinity and a father who partly fits the emasculated role assigned him and partly rebels from it. The vacuum plus the inconsistency of role prevent any true stability in the family structure. Perhaps, if Mr. B. were more totally accepting of the role his wife would assign him, the family would be more stable and perhaps also more distorted in their personality patterns. The nuclear problem might be resolved if Mr. B. could assume the role of dominant and just father, but this does not seem within his present capability.

Before summarizing, some qualifying comments regarding the interpretative significance of non-verbal expressions should be mentioned. These non-verbal cues seem generally to derive from motivations which are less conscious than do verbal expressions, and they are therefore relatively less subject to deliberate control. Nevertheless, non-verbal cues may also to some extent be used in a defensive and perhaps deceptive sense. Sam responds to his mother's gesture of touching him on the shoulder (Item 247) as if it were a manipulative and controlling action, and this type of non-verbal behavior can be as contrived as any verbal expression. Non-verbal behavior may dramatize, deceive, disguise, express or betray; and each expression must be evaluated accordingly.

Also, the hypothesis positing an inverse relation between verbal and non-verbal expressions most likely obtains mainly in reference to verbalizations which are ineffective and fail to express true feeling. Non-verbal expressions must be judged in the context of the total family structure and alongside of verbal communications. They must not be judged solely in isolation but rather in the total context of which they are a part.

Summary

(1) Non-verbal expressions tend to occur in inverse proportion to verbal expressions which are ineffective or fail to express true feeling. Family members who suppress their opinions tend to give vent to more non-verbal forms of expression than do family members who express themselves more fully in words.

(2) Non-verbal expressions may give clues to attitudes or traits which are directly contradictory to expressed opinions. Thus, if the therapist is guided solely by verbalized responses, he may often miss the crux of what is occurring

in therapy.

(3) The non-verbal expressions tend to act as hidden cues whereby the total family is prompted continually to re-enact miniature episodes of shared emotional conflict. This re-enactment of crucial role conflicts may have a cathartic effect and seems oriented toward discharge of accumulated tension. However, its perseverative quality reveals a helpless, repetitive aspect that requires therapeutic intervention.

(4) The therapist elicits suppressed opinions and attitudes of family members by direct challenge and confrontation of preconscious material. In addition, he may pay particular attention to non-verbal expressions, and by calling attention to them be able to reach and formulate some central aspects of the dramatic conflict of the family.

References

1. Ackerman, N.W., The Psychodynamics of Family Life, New York, Basic Books, 1958.
2. Ackerman, N.W., "Prejudicial Scapegoating and Neutralizing Forces in the Family Group, with Special Reference to the Role of 'Family Healer'," Mimeo, 1962.
3. Bateson, G., Jackson, D.D., Haley, J. and Weakland, J., "Toward a Theory of Schizophrenia," Behav. Sci., 1, 251-264, 1956.
4. Birdwhistell, R.L., "Kinesics Analysis in the Investigation of the Emotions," Address to the A.A.A.S., Dec. 1960, Mimeo.
5. Ehrenwald, J., Neurosis in the Family and Patterns of Psychosocial Defense, New York, Hoeber, 1963.
6. Landis, C. and Hunt, W.A., The Startle Pattern, New York, Farrar and Rinehart, 1939.
7. Pittenger, R.E., Hockett, C.F. and Danehy, J.J., The First Five Minutes: A Sample of Microscopic Analysis, Ithaca, New York, Paul Martineau, 1960.

8. Reik, T., Listening with the Third Ear, New York, Farrar, Straus & Co., 1948.

9. Ruesch, J., Therapeutic Communication, New York, Norton, 1961.

10. Schroeder, T., "Psycho-therapeutics: From Art to Science," Psychoanal. Rev., 18, 37-56, 1931.

11. Sherman, M.H., "Peripheral Cues and the Invisible Countertransference," Amer. J. Psychother., to be published.

12. Weakland, J., "The 'Double-Bind' Hypothesis of Schizophrenia and Three-Party Interaction," in Jackson, D.D. (ed.) The Etiology of Schizophrenia, Basic Books, 1960, p. 373-388.

20. A Family Therapist Looks At "Little Hans"

by Herbert S. Strean

From Family Process, vol. 6, no. 2, Sept. 1967. Reprinted by permission.

One of the classics of psychoanalysis is the story of "Little Hans." Hans, a five-year old boy, was so paralyzed by his phobia of horses that he was forced to stay at home and not risk going outdoors for fear that he would be confronted by the animals. His father, a student of Sigmund Freud, decided that he would attempt to rid Hans of his phobia by utilizing the prescribed interpretive interventions of classical psychoanalytic technique developed by Freud for the psychotherapy of neurotics. Under Dr. Freud's guidance, the father met with Hans almost daily over a period of a few months and explained to the boy the reasons for his fear. Little Hans was told that his phobia emanated from his oedipal wishes--his strong erotic attachment to his mother coupled with his wish to displace his father and penetrate mother with his own "widdler." Because Hans was convinced that his sexual desires towards mother and competitive drives towards father were taboo, he had to pay a penalty, namely, castration at the hands of his father. Unable to cope with his strong ambivalence towards his father, Hans repressed the hateful feelings, displaced them on to horses and then feared the horses' hostile retaliation rather than that of his father.

Hans' recovery, according to Freud, was due to the boy's assimilation and integration of his father's interpretations which were mainly focused on Hans' oedipal difficulties. Recognizing that his father would not punish him for his libidinal and aggressive wishes, Hans was free to resume his energetic life outdoors and enter areas where he previously feared to tread (3).

The case of Little Hans has remained a classic; not only has it been utilized to demonstrate the metapsychology of anxiety hysteria, but it reveals poignantly the universal oedipal struggle which all children are alleged to experience. In addition, the case has provided a colorful means of attempting to understand how psychoanalytic interpretations may lead to the uncovering and overcoming of a neurosis, particularly a childhood neurosis.

While studying Little Hans, this writer has, both as a student and as a teacher, either been asked or asked of himself several questions pertinent to the dynamic diagnosis and treatment of this little boy. These questions Freud apparently did not answer in his otherwise brilliant and stimulating treatise. "If the oedipus complex is universal, what is uniquely transpiring in this boy's life that can only be 'compromised' by the development of a paralyzing phobia?" is a query asked by many social work students. The treatment-oriented worker has often inquired, "What is involved in the 'transference' relationship of this boy to his father that induces Hans to accept virtually all of his father's interpretations?" Closely related to this last question is, "Given the ambivalent relationship that Hans had towards his father, why isn't he ambivalent towards his father as a therapist and why doesn't he respond to his therapeutic sessions ambivalently?"

Child guidance workers have pondered the influence of the parents' contemplated divorce on Hans' psychosocial development and on the unfolding of his treatment. "Does not a disturbed marital relationship exacerbate a boy's oedipal difficulties?" is the most often repeated query. Other questions related to familial dynamics are the following: "When Hans' mother threatened the boy that his "widdler" would fall off because of his masturbating, hasn't she indirectly presented some of her own feelings about the penis and about men in general?" "Could not her sexual attitudes possibly imply a disturbed sexual relationship with her husband, reflecting her own feelings of castration and a wish to castrate?"

With the family now more often the unit of diagnosis and treatment in social agencies, clinics, and in the work of some private practitioners, family oriented workers using the Little Hans case as a learning instrument have asked questions like these: "When father enacts the role of therapist and mother is left out of the treatment plan entirely, what does this do to the family's homeostatic balance?" "Isn't father keeping mother away from the 'therapy' and possibly using the child as a weapon against mother?" "What would have happened if mother and father agreed in advance on what to say to Little Hans and presented the 'interpretations' together?"

Just as Freud's case studies of Dora and the Wolf Man have been reevaluated in the light of new understanding and the development of new theory, so too with the increments of knowledge that family oriented therapists now possess it may be possible to refine and enrich our understanding of the case of Little Hans, considered by some as the first family oriented child guidance case in therapeutic history. Buttressed by the findings of the social sciences and ego psychology, impressed with failures in individual therapy, particularly in child guidance treatment when only the child had been involved, and aware that post hospitalization recovery in mental illness has much more to do with the locus of the patient's residence and with whom he eventually interacts than with his diagnosis and prognosis, increasing numbers of professional workers embracing several disciplines are subscribing to a family oriented approach. The family, as currently viewed by many professionals, is a social system with several interacting parts and is governed by the principles of transaction, stability, and the communication of information (4, 5, 6). When the family is viewed as a social system, it is contended that a change in one family member will modify the role interactions and transactions of the others.

As Ackerman (1), Haley (4, 5), Jackson (6), and others have reiterated, the patient with symptoms is not only serving a complex function for the family through his expression of pathology, he is also satisfying the needs of family members by serving what Ackerman has referred to as a "scapegoat function" (1). As the displayed expression of family conflict, the patient is "holding the family together and providing a focus for its discontent" (4). Further, theorists on family dynamics suggest that when the family member with the presenting problem improves, other family members exhibit distress and the dissolution of the family unit is threatened (2, 4, 9).

Referring to the oedipus complex and its vicissitudes in connection with family interaction, Haley has stated:

> . . . the permutations of such a triangle when seen as an actual situation are many, and the child raised in one kind of habitual triangular pattern will presumably learn to behave differently from one raised in a different one, even though the problem of such a triangle is universal (4).

The family oriented practitioner assessing the case of Little Hans would therefore examine it not only from the vantage point of the presenting problem; he would hold as axiomatic that the behavior of one individual in a family exerts influence upon other family members and that a change in one member's behavior provokes responses in the others. Consequently, the family therapist would be interested in the interactions and transactions of Little Hans vis à vis his father and mother as individuals, Hans' perceptions of their marital relationship, the marital relationship itself, and the interdependence of the parent-child, parent-parent, and spouse-spouse subsystems. If we view Hans' family as a gestalt, we will then not only analyze Hans' oedipal fantasies but also attempt to understand what impact his parents had on their development. We would also wish to ascertain what conflicts Hans' oedipal preoccupations induced in his parents and into their marital subsystem.

Children's developmental problems activate unresolved childhood conflicts of their parents so that when a parent seeks assistance from a therapist in relation to his child, he is also presenting a part of himself which seeks help (2, 7, 8, 9). When Hans' father went to Freud, he may have been unconsciously communicating that "I, Hans' father, have oedipal difficulties of my own which I can't resolve. They are being stimulated constantly by my son. Please help me!" It is of interest that concurrent with Hans' developing sexual curiosity, we find his father curious about the sexual theories of Freud and attending his lectures on sex. Papa, in effect, was attempting to get sexual instruction from Freud both in a group and in individual sessions. Based on his quests for sexual information through the media of lectures, individual guidance, and the literature, one may reasonably speculate that the father was having some sexual difficulties of his own.

If our hypothesis concerning the sexual difficulties

that Father was experiencing with his wife is correct, and if we consider the dearth of communication that transpired between the mother and father throughout the case, it would follow that Hans' sexual curiosity could not be discussed by Mama and Papa together, either with or without Hans present. Apparently, Hans' burgeoning sexual curiosity and attendant fantasies induced considerable anxiety in both parents and in turn, exacerbated their withdrawal from each other. Intensified were Hans' erotic desires towards Mother because he sensed an increased availability of her by virtue of father's withdrawal from her. Furthermore, Father, who attended lectures on sex in his spare time and did not spend very much time with his wife, emerged throughout the story as a tender, maternal man, one whose lack of aggressiveness could only strengthen a boy's oedipal guilt. Hence, Papa and Mama avoided each other, avoided discussing sexual questions about Hans with each other, and interestingly, Hans developed a symptom which had as its major feature, avoidance. Because there was a dearth of verbal communication in the interdependent triangular relationship on sex, Hans squelched his feelings and thoughts on the subject and displaced his conflicts on to an object that could not verbally communicate at all, namely, a horse.

Freud, who saw nine or ten patients a day and then burned the midnight oil writing up his notes and studying them, could have felt a strong indentification with Hans' father--both men were fascinated by the sexual theories on children but neither of them had, in all probability, an active adult sexual life. Perhaps Freud chose not to see the problem that Hans' father presented as evolving from the latter's inner distress because Freud, like the father, wished to forget about adult sexuality for himself. Therefore, we can view Hans as displacing his conflict on to horses, the father displacing his sexual conflict on to the childhood sexual theories of Freud, and Freud displacing the therapeutic task before him on to supplying the father with "horse sense" on children.

The relationship between Hans' father and Freud became recapitulated in the father's treatment of Hans; childhood sexuality was again the topic of discussion. Since these therapeutic encounters transpired almost daily, we can tentatively conclude that the sexual discussions provided both partners with some sexual stimulation and gratification.

Father and son, in effect, were having almost daily verbal sexual intercourse and excluding the mother. As Freud, himself, has taught us, when an oedipal conflict in a boy is strong, a common defense is to repress his competitive aggression toward the father and deny the love attachment towards the mother. The boy then submits to Father in a homosexual manner, his hostility goes underground, and a love and beloved relationship between father and son is formed. Father's sexual talks with Hans apparently seduced the boy into a submissive relationship with him, and Hans became more and more positively suggestible to his father's interpretations. To please his father, Hans gave up the fear of horses, which was Father's main objective. It will be recalled that as the case material unfolded, and not prior to the therapy, Hans became increasingly effeminate and submissive. He began to have fantasies of becoming a woman and dreamed that he had given birth to a baby. Like his mother who had given birth to Hans' baby sister during his pre-oedipal phase, Hans became, psychologically, his father's wife and surrendered his own virility.

As we know, Mother was excluded and probably excluded herself from the consultations with Freud. She did not attend Freud's lectures on sex and was totally uninvolved in the treatment of her son. Is there a possibility that the rage she felt in being a loner was conveyed to Hans when she admonished him for his masturbatory activity (which is performed alone) by threatening him with the loss of his "widdler"? Further, as Mother was excluded she probably excluded and no doubt aided and abetted the intensification of Father and Hans' homosexual attraction.

As family therapists have demonstrated, when the family member with the presenting problem improves, other family members exhibit distress and/or the family unit can possibly be threatened with dissolution (5). Hans' phobia was the displayed expression of family conflict and held the family together, preserving its equilibrium. When Hans, the family member with the presenting problem, improved, the parents' marriage soon after was dissolved. The mutual avoidance pattern of both parents towards each other reinforced Father's attachment to his son wherein Hans became his father's wife. As Mother became further alienated from her husband and son (and eventually bowed out entirely), Hans and his father drew closer. Father evolved into both a mother and father for Hans, was ascribed strong omnipotence by the latter, and the patient was cured through love. Hans, in his submission to Father, complied with his father's prescription that was received from Freud, namely, that "the phobia is nonsense and ridiculous to keep" (3).

The set of events that transpired in the treatment of Hans occurs frequently in current casework treatment and psychotherapy, particularly in the treatment of marital partners. One spouse forms a love and beloved relationship with the therapist--the latter becomes the most important person in the client's life--and the alienated spouse, no longer the loved object, withdraws further. Like Hans, who esteemed and idealized his therapist, many patients do likewise with their treatment partners who become psychological spouses for them. Hence, there is a certain truth in the allegations levelled at various forms of treatment by the laity when they exclaim that "psychiatry makes the patient get a divorce." As in the treatment of Hans where most of the boy's aggression went underground and little of it was cathected towards this therapist, many patients and therapists form a pact which is to "love, honor and obey"; the patient's spouse is either attacked by them in the therapy or else forgotten completely.

If Freud had adhered to the well proven child guidance axiom that the child and his functioning are expressions of the parents' egos, rather than giving Hans' father advice and sexual information, he would have "begun where the client was" (2) and explored the significance of the father's request. The results of the treatment might have been different if Father's underlying need behind his request was responded to with real therapeutic understanding; his marital and sexual relationship with his wife could have eventually become the therapeutic focus. If he had been treated as a client in his own right, Father, instead of recapitulating with Hans the kind of tête à tête he experienced with Freud, could have emerged as more of a husband and sexual partner of his wife. This might have modified Little Hans' perception of his father and mother and could have influenced his oedipal situation for the better. By the demonstration of more mature and more differentiated sexual roles in real life situations, Father and Mother might have helped Hans come to more of a resolution of his oedipal difficulties than he did through his stimulating sex talks with his father. A discussion of Father's own sexual problems would probably have made Mother a subject or object of treatment and a different oedipal milieu would have been created for the boy.

At the end of Freud's exposition on Little Hans, there is a postscript describing a meeting with Hans several years after the therapy had terminated, when Hans was 19. Freud's impression of Hans was that the latter had grown to be a vigorous young man free from the phobia of horses. There is no report on Hans' current sexual adjustment, but there is a statement from Hans to Freud that both his parents were remarried after their divorce and that Hans was living alone (3). Freud did not venture to assess the desirability or impact of this living arrangement on Hans. Of definite interest to the family therapist is that the three members of the system all went their separate ways. The phobic symptom had "held the family together and provided a focus for its discontent" and "when the family member with the presenting problem improved, the family unit was threatened with dissolution" (4). In Hans' case, the family was not only threatened with dissolution when the phobia was dissolved, but it actually happened; each of the three members eventually removed themselves from each other.

As family therapists, we have observed in Little Hans an excellent illustration of how a symptom of one member binds and protects a whole family constellation. It enriches our understanding of the protective and defensive quality of symptoms and how their premature removal can intensify interpersonal difficulties rather than diminish them. Important for all therapists is to study the defensive needs of a patient or patients and to comprehend the necessity for the maintenance of symptoms, for they often protect and sustain the family. Only when the total family system appreciates the symptom as an expression of the "family symptom" does it have a real chance for a healthy resolution.

References

1. Ackerman, N.W., _The Psychodynamics of Family Life, New York, Basic Books, 1958._

2. Feldman, Y., "A Casework Approach Toward Understanding Parents of Emotionally Disturbed Children," _Social Work,_ 3, 23-29, 1958.

3. Freud, S., "Analysis of a Phobia in a Five Year Old Boy," Collected Papers, 3, New York, Basic Books, 1959.

4. Haley, J., Strategies of Psychotherapy, New York, Grune and Stratton, 1963.

5. Haley, J., "Whither Family Therapy," Fam. Proc., 1, 69-100, 1962.

6. Jackson, D.D., "The Question of Family Homeostasis," Psychiat. Quart., 31, 79-90, 1957.

7. Rangell, L., "The Analysis of a Doll Phobia," The Yearbook of Psychoanal., 9, 178-198, New York, International Universities Press, 1953.

8. Strean, H., "Treating Parents of Emotionally Disturbed Children Through Role Playing," Psychoan. and Psychan. Rev., 47, 67-75, 1960.

9. Strean, H.S., "Treatment of Mothers and Sons in the Absence of the Father," Social Work, 6, 29-35, 1961.

10. Wolpe, J. and Rachman, S., "Psychoanalytic Evidence: A Critique Based on Freud's case of 'Little Hans'," J. of Nervous and Mental Diseases, 131, 135-148, 1960.

Part IV

The Social System

21. Social Work with Retardates in Their Social Systems

by Leonard N. Brown

Reprinted by permission from Mental Retardation, vol. 5, no. 3, June 1967, p. 17-20, a publication of the American Association on Mental Deficiency.

All persons occupy various positions or statuses in society. As they interact together around some common purpose, and as these interactions are repeated in similar social situations, a pattern of relationships develops. The behaviors of the participants within these social exchanges are roles or norms of how to act. The social system is this pattern of relationships among people where there are expectations of behavior that guide the interaction.

In large measure, a person acts on the basis of what he thinks is expected of him within his reference groups. He responds not only to the other person but to the social situation in which the transaction takes place. The social situation itself has certain expectations of appropriate behavior. Our role performance enables us to make some predictions about what our behavior will mean to ourselves through the reactions of other people. It is a means of developing greater stability in our lives. We fashion our activity to be consistent with the patterns of role expectation which we have learned over time. Since the parts or roles of the system are interrelated and interdependent, a change in one part will affect the entire system.

The retardate often has difficulty which appropriate role behavior. His social contacts and development may be limited. There are less opportunities for him to participate in a wide range of social situations. To some extent he is unable to perform adequately because of his intellectual deficit. However, he often faces restrictions beyond necessity because persons may not be comfortable in knowing how to act with a retarded person. This lack of opportunities within the community increases the social disability of the person with mental retardation. He may be uncertain about the kind of behavior that is socially acceptable since the recognition of approval for his actions may not be forthcoming. After repeated signs of disapproval, he may withdraw from attempting the behavior again.

In social work with the mentally retarded it is especially important that the retardate receive help in relation to the social systems that are significant in his life. It is through his interaction within these social systems that his social behavior finds expression. Since this is a transactional arrangement, with parts of the system contributing to each other, one part that is strengthened will have a positive influence on the other. For the purposes of this article, the client system in social work will be considered as any combination of persons within a social system that occupy a position of receiving social services. A helping system, on the other hand, presupposes some willingness of these persons to participate in mutual helping relationships with the social worker.

The Helping System

In this approach to practice, the social worker may start with the individual, small group or larger social system itself as the client system. Through the social worker's exploration of needs and problems with the initial client system, a beginning boundary of relationships is identified as being important influences on the client system. For the adolescent who is mildly retarded and living at an institution, the important relationships would most likely be with persons who have some responsibility for his care and development. This would include his peers, and those in the training and clinical services. Assuming there is still contact with the home, the family would be another strong influence in the lives of the residents.

As these relevant persons become more aware of the retardate's needs and problems, they may be more able to assume a nurturing role and become more explicit regarding their expectations of his behavior. In this way it is more possible for him to learn appropriate role behavior which will bring satisfactions in the course of his interactions within these social systems. At the same time, the retardate is encouraged to make known his expectations of others so that he may be more responsibe to their needs. Through this process of communication, some common understandings may develop which will support the clarity of reciprocal role relationships.

The participation of significant persons in the life of the retarded individual will depend on the willingness of the retardate to involve others and the accessibility and priority of persons who have the potential for assuming this nurturing position. As we are able to foster this kind of positive social climate, these helping relationships become more possible. The structures in which these relationships exist, such as the home situation or the institutional services, may be lacking in promoting opportunities for social growth. The rehabilitation process often includes a rearrangement of services or the creation of new services to meet these needs. A social systems approach would direct intervention at the system itself so that the reciprocal-role relationships within the system can be more therapeutic.

The interaction within the client system creates strains that often result from subgroup power conflicts and clashing roles. These strains may represent distortions and incompleteness within parts of the client system or in relationships between systems. It is natural for these tensions to exist as a result of differences in the way people react to one another. These differences may be healthy or unhealthy, depending on whether they free or block further exchange among the persons involved. Distortions or misconceptions of actual happenings may inhibit an honest display of difference, leading to the need for clarification. The idea of "clarification" is contained in the general formulation that a major function of the social worker with the group is to reflect the meaning of behavior in the social reality of the group. Through client involvement by the social worker in considering the meaning of these conflict situations, as well as in the development of commonly perceived goals, the individuals and subgroups are better able to express contrary views and develop more understanding of how the system relationships can be more helpful for the client system members.

A Student Program

I would like to describe here an approach to social work practice that attempts to support these contentions. The practitioners, in this case, were second-year graduate students in social work, with concentrations in social group work and social casework. They were part of a unit of eight students, which included a field instructor in each method. The project was supported by a training grant from the Vocational Rehabilitation Administration. The setting was the E. R. Johnstone Training and Research Center, Bordentown, New Jersey, a state institution and rehabilitation center for 300 adolescent boys and girls who are mildly and moderately retarded. The residents all have varying degrees of social and emotional problems. The population comes from other state institutions for the mentally retarded and some come directly from the community. Social service is available to residents and their parents through individual interviews and group sessions. Additional clinical services include psychological counseling and testing, speech and hearing therapy, and medical and psychiatric services.

The adolescents are all considered students, since they are involved in an active academic and vocational training program. Campus recreation is provided during the leisure time hours. Those under 16 years of age are generally in a full-time academic program. The older students are advanced through on-campus and off-campus training, as indicated by their progress. The residents are returned to the community as soon as they show some capability for making a satisfactory adjustment within their own home, in foster placement, or in an independent or sheltered work situation.

The learning experiences, which flow from the assessment and intervention within social systems, include a wide range of social work activities with social systems which are relevant to the residents. Besides the retardates themselves, these include the attendants, the social service staff, the institutional administration, the community and the families. As there can be mutual helping relationships developed between these systems and the retardates, and clear role expectations within each of these systems which do not conflict with each other, it is assumed that both the retardates and their "significant others" will be more functional for each other. This is known as the process of systemic linkage, whereby two systems may on some occasions act as one, and the goals of the systems become more similar. Systemic linkage presupposes some interaction of the system around a purpose. This kind of engagement leads to norms and sentiments which make it more possible for the systems to act in the interests of each other.

The Method

In the assignment which describes this practice, two social work students were given responsibility for a particular section of one of the cottages housing 14 adolescents. One of the purposes of this assignment was to develop a therapeutic milieu. Their first task was to select residents for this living area and they did so on the basis of four criteria. These included the following: (1) the adolescents were in the educable range of retardation, (2) their parents were interested and accessible for social service, (3) there was evidence of a need for social service, and (4) they were able to return to the community and be placed in a work situation.

The attendants chosen for this special project had or could learn therapeutic attitudes. The social system analysis within this part of the cottage led to an understanding of the resident's interests and concerns, status-roles of participants, position of subgroupings and norms of behavior.

The adolescents were all seen in one of two small groups that met weekly with a social worker. (Social worker and social work student will be used synonymously.) Inasmuch as possible, the boys were grouped with their friends. Some of the adolescents were also seen individually as it seemed appropriate. In addition, the social worker met with representatives of both small groups and the attendant to plan a group program that would involve all 14 boys. The program made use of activity and discussion on the needs and problems of their group living situation. During this time the attendant worked together with the social worker. The attendant made use of some of his particular skills, such as teaching acrobatics, to create a closer bond with the residents.

A family night, including the parents and children within the project, was held monthly. During this time the parents participated in a group discussion of their immediate interests and concerns and then took part in a joint activity with their children, such as square dancing or bingo. This was followed by refreshments for all the families. At the time of the parent discussions the adolescents were in another part of the large room where they were involved in group activity with another social worker. When it was time for the families to get together after the discussion, the social workers joined with the families on an informal basis for further discussions and activity.

Besides the monthly family meetings, some of these same parents met for group discussions on a regular basis at another time during the month. Some of the parents were also seen individually on specific requests for help. An important phase of the program included weekly conferences or team meetings with the attendants and other members of the clinical or training staff who may have been seeing these same adolescents. Since this program was innovative and had implications for changes throughout social service, the director of social service was also present. A social worker chaired these meetings and wrote minutes which were distributed to the administrative staff and department heads of the clinical and training services. In this way there was communication to the services which also had responsibility for the residents, and to the administration, who would be in a position to make whatever structural changes might be therapeutically desirable on a more permanent basis.

The social workers often made informal visits to the unit in order to observe and meet with the adolescents within their natural subgroups. These additional informal visits provided the adolescents with a further access to the social workers, who were also in a better position to understand the effects of the total living situation on the behavior of the resident. Besides meeting with the groups within the institution, the social worker often made trips into the community and made use of community facilities, including the local YMCA, the bowling alley, the miniature golf range, parks, stores and eating places. These kinds of activities provided opportunities for the adolescents to make gradual transitions to the community. They were able to discuss these community visits as a group during the time that they were participating in the group experiences.

Family Interaction

What I have just described is social work practice with 14 adolescents and some of the related social systems in their environment. Looking more closely at the retardate, his family and the social worker as a helping system within the context of this project, I believe it is significant that whole families were able to meet together. Very often we find that when we meet with parents only, we learn about their perceptions of what took place in parent-child relationships. The same would be true if we were seeing the children in relation to their parents. It would be the child's perception of the child-parent relationship that would be presented as reality. In the type of situation which I have described, the parents and children are in the same room together. When a parent talks about her child the other parents in the group are able to recognize the child from their own observations and experiences with him in the course of their interaction together. In this way the distortions that often result from misperceptions of another person are minimized as other parents are able to contribute their own observations of the parent-child relationship. Through this process, it is more likely that the focus of discussion within the parent's group will be on the quality of the interaction itself rather than with only one party in the transaction.

Another important feature of this type of structural arrangement is that the families are able to interact with each other around the common purpose of participating together as a family, creating identification with the family as a functioning unit. As the families are able to have fun together through their joint participation in activities of their choice, the parents and children have a further opportunity to see each other in a more favorable light. The child can see and feel that his parent is in a more relaxed, amiable frame of mind and the parent, in turn, is able to react more positively to his child. In this type of engagement the parents and children may be able to develop new and more satisfying patterns of behavior with each other. The parent may be finding more gratification in his role as parent. Being separated from the child often brings some feelings of guilt on the part of the parents, and coming to the institution and participating with the child in a series of satisfying experiences can provide the parent with a sense of greater fulfillment in his nurturing role.

As the families were able to meet together over a period of time, the cohesiveness within the group began to develop and grow stronger. Parents were able to discuss some of their feelings about being separated from their children. They were also able to plan together what they wanted to do. For instance, the parents group began to want to do more for and with their children. This led to some exploratory meetings with the institutional administration, and, as a result, the parents took part in decorating the rooms of the adolescents, with the help of their children. In addition to regular meetings, the families planned trips together outside the institution. They had picnics, went to the circus and engaged in sports activities. The parents were able to observe and participate with each other in the care of their children. A parent is sometimes able to notice differences in the way other parents respond to his child, leading to further self-examination of his own relationship with his child. It is often easier to act as a "good" parent with someone else's child. In such a case, the parent is somewhat freed from the emotional entanglements of his own parent-child relationship. The child is also able to have relationships with adults other than his parents, but acting in a parental role. In the traditional parent discussion group, parents often know the "right" thing to say about how they should act toward their child. They are expounding the role of the parent as they would like it to be. In the situation described here, they actually have the opportunity to test out this behavior and learn new ways of achieving the desired role of parent. Parents and children are able to support each other in their new ways and relating to each other. The norms that develop through the multiple interaction might approximate a more normal parental role.

In addition to contributing to the rehabilitation process within the institution, this type of family centered program was actually helping both the parents and the children in preparation for the child's return to the home. Because the social workers were able to become part of this process, they were able to help clarify some of the differences within the family. The children and parents were able to find ways of communicating with one another so that understanding of how each one could contribute to the family became more possible, and differences became more explicit. The interaction by the families with the institutional administration led to increased institutional responsiveness to the families' needs and some restructuring of services to meet these needs. The therapeutic milieu which was developed within this section of the cottage had an effect on the total institution. Needless to say, this kind of assignment provided many enriching learning experiences for the graduate students of social work. They were able not only to understand and provide services to the adolescent and his parents separately but also to use themselves within the interactional process of the family, and the families in relation to the institution.

In this description of practice, there were various arrangements of client systems. The initial client system was the cottage section of 14 boys and those persons directly responsible for their care, such as the cottage personnel and the social workers. As the client system explored together their needs and problems, there was an attempt to reach a common therapeutic purpose. The process of this exploration enables persons within the client system to become more aware of how they can contribute to each other. If and when other persons are recognized as being influential in the social functioning of the client system, such as the family in the practice illustration, the client system may attempt to involve these individuals in the helping process. When the family and "significant others" are able to understand the purpose of their involvement and agree to participate, they become part of a helping system. As there continues to be involvement with relevant persons in mutual helping efforts, the process of systemic linkage is enhanced and a more total therapeutic milieu is possible.

Conclusion

In conclusion, I have attempted to point out how the study of social systems enables the practitioner to understand the individual, family, social group and organization as interrelated and interdependent. In the systemic view of social work, the social work student intervenes within a variety of associated social systems. He is able to understand behavior as a manifestation of the way these systems connect with each other. Social work practice is directed at these intersystem relationships, both within the group and with the group in relation to its environment.

With a common body of knowledge about systems of varying complexities, the practitioner may be able to develop ways of being helpful within a wide variety of social situations. The knowledge and understanding of social systems seems to have implications for all of social work practice. It may be one of the ways that we will be able to conceptualize and practice a social work method, with services to individuals, groups and communities in relation to the social systems of which they are a part.

22. Understanding and Working with Alienated and Rebellious Youth

by William Neal Brown

Paper presented at 61st Annual State Conference on Probation, Grossinger's, Grossinger, New York, Oct. 7, 1969.

Here sits enigma--sharp averted eyes,
Half slouched, half tensed, and almost violent grace.
Only his hands reveal how much he tries
to keep on showing 'nothing' in his face.
The statement of complaint, police reports,
These are the known, the outward surface acts.
I ask the routine questions, note retorts,
and watch the mouth that wants to stick to facts.
Tomorrow I will meet his folks, his street,
Attempt to find the threads to the design,
Seek out the loom, though warped and incomplete,
And strive to keep the pattern his, not mine.
I cannot walk in his distorted land,
Just look across, and try to understand.[1]

In an earlier published paper,[2] the writer has commented on the alienation of youth in our society, and some of the factors that make for alienation. The factors discussed there were: (1) the trend toward urbanization, (2) the egalitarian thrust, (3) the drive to "succeed", (4) the concept of "fit", and (5) the absence of "caring."[2] The sense of that piece was to the effect of organizational and structural realities of our time on a sense of being left out or alienated on the part of youth. This paper now attempts to deal with some of the effects of alienation as they have implication for probation officers in understanding and working with delinquent youth.

It should be noted that the word "delinquency" is a vague and imprecise term. For this reason there are those who claim the study of delinquency to be so arbitrary as to be useless. For the purpose of this paper, delinquency will be defined as those acts which violate duly established laws and so result in some form of adjudication of the act. Youngsters whose behavior falls in this category are the ones who come to the attention of probation officers. They are the subjects of this discussion.

The difficulties of the adolescent period of the life cycle are well documented both in the literature and in our own observation.[3] Most probation officers are aware of the physical phenomena that characterize this period--the resurgence of physical growth, the development of parts of the body heretofore dormant, and the beginning of glandular secretions that determine sexual balance. Most of us are familiar with the struggle with ego-identity and the resultant identity diffusion of the adolescent.[4] He is searching for the answer in the question: "Who am I?", in terms of sexual identity, vocational potential, and social relationships. The period is marked by fluctuations and unpredictability occasioned by the ambivalent thrust toward adult independence and the simultaneous pull toward childhood dependence and security. The high priority given to peer associations and the competition with and disparagement of the parent of the same sex are familiar benchmarks. Adolescence is a difficult period for any growing person. These difficulties are compounded for that deviant person whom we describe as a "juvenile delinquent."

Much has been written about the "culture of poverty."[5] One could just as easily refer to a "culture of delinquency." It needs be noted, however, that the reason this is so is largely conditioned by our professional responses to social stratification and the way that delinquency is defined so that certain individuals are both arrested and adjudicated delinquent more often than are others. The social correlates of arrest, for example, are: 1) age, 2) sex, 3) race, 4) place of residence, and 5) socio-economic status. Ergo: For a person to be arrested in this society, he is:

3 times as likely to be under 25
10 times as likely to be a man rather than a woman

> Negroes, three times more frequently than whites He is more likely to live in the center city and to be of low occupational status--low education, low income.[6]

Because of the variations that exist in how social mores are applied and enforced, it is difficult to know just how pervasive are the acts which come under the rubric of "juvenile delinquency." We do know that the preponderance of those apprehended and adjudicated as delinquent are those who commit relatively serious property crimes--burglary, larceny, and motor vehicle theft, and crimes against the person--mugging, rape, and criminal assault--which are more prevalent in lower class districts.[7] Thus, there is a remarkably high correlation between the "culture of poverty" and the "culture of delinquency."

Poor people living in an urban setting share several universal characteristics. These include such factors as inadequate income (living on a level well below that which is possible and average for the community).[8] It also includes frequent unemployment or employment in unskilled seasonal jobs, minimal education, and living in slums in sub-standard housing with many persons to a room. Often, it means inadequate nutrition, with resulting health problems. It usually means inadequate services and resources to deal with physical and mental problems.[9]

Psychologically, poverty involves a state of mind. It usually carries with it "apathy, inertia, indifference and loss of initiative." It may cause "envy, bitterness, and self-depreciation of the ego," resulting in hostility, anomie, and disturbed role identification.[10] The poor housing and over-crowding influence motivation and self-evaluation, and there is much stress from a constant need to get along with people in cramped quarters. Furthermore, the crowding causes a person to look to others for satisfaction in life, to be cynical about people, to be uninterested in solitary pursuits, and to have an early initiation into sexual behavior. The crowding leads to friction and confusion within the home which causes family members to spend much of their time on the streets. This in turn affects family relationships, parental control, and study habits. Alvin Schorr has stated that from poor housing situations there comes a pessimism, passivity, and a state of dissatisfaction, restlessness, cynicism, and difficulties in childbearing.[11] Stability of family life is affected, since we note that separation, desertion, divorce, and family size vary inversely with income.[12]

The central role of education in upward social and vocational mobility has been amply documented.[13] It is also well documented that the poorer districts have the poorest schools with the poorer teachers, higher teacher turnover, and less adequate facilities.[14] This has numerous repercussions on the youth of the community who find school dull, teachers non-stimulating. Thus, lower class students are not motivated to continue in school. This added to economic factors which pressure them to be employed as soon as possible, and the institutionalized devaluation of school in the lower class homes, makes school dropout a considerable problem in lower class areas (average 70-80% there as compared with 40% for the population as a whole.)[15] Armed with little education and that of poor quality, many of these lower class children enter the vocational world unequipped to get a meaningful job; or, in some instances, even to get a job at all. The resultant sporadic employment or unemployment serves to reinforce the hopelessness, cynicism, and apathy already in his home life, as well as his self-image of inadequacy. It is easy to see that these lower class youth have minimal chance for "success" along the expected, socially accepted routes. This being precluded, they become delinquent and seek the standard ends of success --recognition, status, reward--but through deviant means.

It would seem to be important for the probation officer to be aware of the internal and external pressures that operate on delinquent youth. By and large, they come from families that have more than their share of social problems --low level of employment or unemployment, family disintegration, illegitimacy, and a high adult and juvenile crime rate. Many of the youth of this group are from "broken homes" with one or both parents missing.[16]

The officer should be aware of the latent value placed on aggression. It may seem strange to categorize "aggression" as a value. However, to an economically and socially deprived group, aggression becomes a value of high rank. Sometimes it is veiled, surreptitious and devious; it is quite often unconscious and practically always unspoken; but, somehow, it comes to be right to "take," to "force" that which one is denied legitimately, by circuitous and often illegitimate means.[17]

The officer who would work in a rehabilitative way with hostile and alienated youth must take into account some cultural issues which plague correctional practice. Among these is a rather widespread, if not universal, tendency for the general public to perceive probation as essentially and primarily punitive rather than rehabilitative. (This notwithstanding the term corrections which is intended to imply reform or rehabilitation.) In addition, there is a clash in values between concern for individuals and pressure for conformance to group standards and requirements; the concern of society for results more than the meaning of experiences to individuals. As an overlay to these generalized cultural characteristics, the special characteristics of a correctional system with its requirements of structure, restraint, authority, and control must be taken into account in assessing the rehabilitative task.

Foremost, in his approach to the hostile adolescent, the probation officer must assess his own social and cultural background and how wide the gap between his life experience and that of the offender. How can he bridge this gap in such a way that meaningful communication and relationship can be established? As he makes this assessment, the officer is most likely to find that simply because he was (and is) a part of the larger culture, unless he develops considerable self-understanding, he will be quite hindered in trying to develop an integrated understanding of the people he wants to help. Professionally, this difficulty is referred to as acting on the basis of stereotypic perception, i.e. acting on the basis of a stereotype derived from acculturation in terms of "the criminal," "the offender," "the in-mate," "the juvenile delinquent." The concept of realistic self-acceptance and self-understanding as a basis for understanding and helping others should be a common thread running through the rehabilitative process. The foregoing discussion of socio-cultural influences on both learning and functioning should serve to underscore this point. The probation officer must be alert to his own needs and reactions to authority and dependency, and he must be able to discipline those needs.

Given the kind of "self" and "societal" knowledge here described, one of the most helpful things a probation officer can do for an alienated, hostile youth is to provide him a new and constructive experience with authority. The youth comes to probation with a string of unsuccessful experiences with authority figures--usually an experience of neglect or rejection (or both) on the part of home and school, a punitive experience with arresting and adjudicating officials. By the time he gets to the probation officer, "his back is arched." He feels that nobody cares--and, he doesn't care, either. He reacts to the officer either with passivity and withdrawal, reflecting his alienation, or with hostility, reflecting his aggression. It is at this point that all too many probation officers become blocked by the dilemma of "help" versus "authority," or to put it in correctional terminology, treatment versus surveillance. They seem constantly fearful of being accused of pampering the delinquent. (Or worse, they are blocked from taking the necessary steps toward help by their own reluctance to do what they view as "pampering.")

The successful probation officer knows that "help" and "authority" are not necessarily contradictory concepts. Particularly with the adolescent, he is aware that definitely established and maintained limits are prerequisite to healthy personality development. The individual grows into emotional maturity through reaction to these limits, to the needed authority in his environment. Thus, help and authority must be regarded not as contradictory entities but as complementary facets of the same process. The problem in probation practice is not which to use but how to integrate the use of both realistically.

> Albert T. is a 14-year-old, Negro boy placed on probation following a sexual assault on a 12-year old white boy. The probationer lives in a low cost housing development in a congested neighborhood with his mother and younger brother. His father's whereabouts are unknown. The mother, youthful in appearance and quite attractive, works rather than receive public assistance. Both boys are left largely to their own devices during daylight hours. The probationer's school attendance and performance are sporadic and uneven. At one point early in his probation, he "stole" twenty dollars from his mother's bedside table, taking the money to school to buy candy and notions for his classmates. The probationer's father also has been on probation with the same court; and, at one point served 26 months in the disciplinary barracks in Milwaukee, Wisconsin.

> The mother was hostile and defensive when the probation officer discussed the supervision of the boys, and her apparent rejection of them. "What am I supposed to do? They've got to eat!" She expressed feelings of bitterness, of being imposed on and judged unfairly in the light of the economic pressure under which she struggled. This economic pressure and the constant need to adjust to new and changing sets of circumstances have resulted in an extremely uncertain and unstable life for the boys. (During his eight years of school life, Albert had attended ten different schools.)
>
> In his contacts with the probation officer, Albert showed a lack of spontaneity; he seemed to sulk and was a constant thumbsucker. When he did talk, he was defensive and his tone resentful, antagonistic, and rebellious.

Does this boy need "help" or "authority"? Obviously, he needs both. The probation officer must reach him behind the facade he has erected for his own protection. Somehow, the gaps in this boy's life that have been left by the mother's rejection and the father's absence must be filled. The negative feelings engendered by the kind of life he has lived must be nullified to some degree before Albert is ready to move and deal with the "here and now." He needs considerable "authority," but it has to be an authority that conveys the feeling that the authority is imposed because somebody cares.

Albert must be convinced that the probation officer is really interested in him, that the officer "cares," and truly wants to help. This is not an easy task but neither is it an impossible one. At the simplest level, the two must learn to talk to one another, to communicate. One of the first things that a professional helper learns is that he must start "where the client is." Nowhere is this more true than in the area of language. Where language systems are different, the onus is on the probation officer to find a way to reduce or reconcile the differences so that he may enter into the probationer's "world" and find him "where he is." (And, it can be safely assumed that when an adult deals with an adolescent, there will be differences in the language systems. Moreover, this difference in adult and youthful speech patterns may be further complicated by class and ethnic differences.) The probation officer must learn the language of the world in which the probationer moves, and he must learn to use this language in a way that does not appear stilted or artificial.

Next--in Albert's case--the probationer must perceive some change in his life circumstances that accrues from his contact with probation. The officer has many leads for modifying the environment: What can be done about daytime supervision? School is a real problem for Albert: how can the officer reduce the pressure there? Can a substitute be found to fill the void created by the absence of the father? Before Albert can be expected to "take hold," he must have at least some hope that there is reason for doing so.

There is another important barrier to the giving and receiving of help with which the probation officer must deal. This is the obstacle created by role and status considerations. The social roles of probation officer and probationer combine to form a situation in which supraordinate status is imputed to the one and subordinate to the other. Many people resent the feeling of helplessness, of "lack of control," which this situation engenders. Probationers attempt to minimize this feeling in many different ways. Some attempt to socialize the relationship, to establish a climate of camaraderie which is an effort to negate the role and status differentials in the relationship. Others react with diffuse hostility or other forms of subtle resistance. Whatever the nature of the probationer's response to this aspect of supervision, it must be recognized and dealt with by the officer for it is sure to influence the kind and quality of communication between them. Role and status differentials pose a danger to the officer, too. It is all too easy for the insecure officer to "hide" behind them, to assume a condescending manner, and "talk down" to the probationer. This approach increases the probationer's anxiety about his status and creates more defensiveness and resistance in the process of supervision.

By the very nature of their work together, as a result of the kind of life circumstances that bring them together, there <u>is</u> a difference in the role and status of the officer and the probationer. This fact has to be recognized and accepted by both. On the officer's part, in order to open up the most free channels of communication between them, he must constantly work at reducing the gap caused by this difference, without allowing the relationship to deteriorate to one of "buddies" or of antagonist and protagonist.

Having worked for so many years with probation officers, I can already hear an unspoken question from the audience. It comes in one word: "How?" Let me respond to this question by saying that, in my view, no one can give "chapter and verse," a cookbook type blueprint for dealing with each and every delinquent youth. Each case must be dealt with in terms of its dimensions. Nonetheless, there are some general propositions that should prove useful. It is to those that I would like to direct this discussion.

We are not quite sure of the dynamics of the phenomenon, but professional helpers know that people who are troubled find release in discussing their troubles with a receptive listener. Despite this, there are probation officers who spend disproportionate amounts of valuable supervision time telling, admonishing, and directing the probationer. (One might hypothesize that they secure the same kind of release in this type of activity.) However, this is a sure way to dam up communication. The skillful officer will encourage the probationer to talk and give him ample opportunity to do so. To be sure, the flow of the probationer's production has some direction from the officer, but this direction takes the form of well placed and carefully worded questions. When the probationer has only to listen to the admonitions of the probation officer, the officer has little opportunity to assess his thought processes, his feelings, and his expectations. On the other hand, when the probationer has to respond to questions, he has to struggle to develop a response, he must order his thought processes, and he is forced to an evaluation of his own situation. Quite often, in the midst of such a process, the probationer will pause to acknowledge feelings or relationships of which he had been unaware before, because he had not had this type of struggle to put his own situation in perspective. It is a cliche of the helping professions that the skillful helper is a "good listener"; I would add that he is also a good questioner.

Another way of reaching the probationer is through empathic response. Empathy is often loosely and somewhat simply defined as the capacity to put oneself "in the other fellow's boots." It is differentiated from sympathy, because that term implies pity or condescension. However it is defined, it is much more easily described than actualized. In reality it is extremely difficult to understand the other person's situation and to put oneself figuratively in his place. Much more important, when such understanding is achieved, it rarely lends itself to verbal communication. It is asking a lot to ask a young, unmarried female probation officer to put herself "in the boots" of an unmarried, neglectful mother; or, a young upwardly mobile, middle-class oriented probation officer to understand "the boots" of a delinquent adolescent. Yet, this is what is required for a truly empathic response.

Communication and relationship are enhanced when the officer does understand the situation of the probationer and can convey verbally, in manner, and in other non-verbal responses some understanding of the problems with which the probationer must cope. When this occurs the probationer is freed to discuss his situation in dimensions which would be avoided if he felt the officer could not understand.

Much of what occurs in the communication process between the probation officer and the probationer is non-verbal, or it is tangential or circuitous to the expressed issue at hand. This is similar to cases that come to social agencies where mothers come asking for financial aid or for help with a non-conforming child; when, as the story unfolds, it is clear to the worker that neither of these is really the problem. Rather, a marital problem about which she cannot talk is the problem that needs to be dealt with. For reasons of apprehension or self-protection, people frequently need to communicate at a superficial level. Communication is enhanced when the officer is able to recognize unexpressed problems or concerns that have more bearing on the difficulty of the situation than those which the probationer is expressing. To "cut through" to these latent levels is one of the surest ways of conveying understanding of the situation. Once this has happened--and without catastrophe--the probationer's apprehension is diminished, and he is freed to fully discuss his situation.

Earlier mention has been made of the probation officer's need to reach out to the probationer's language system. When a person is burdened with problems and suffering under the added pressure of a language barrier, nothing is more likely to reduce tension and increase self-esteem than an honest effort on the part of the officer to bridge this barrier, without all of the "giving" being by the probationer. At a point where the officer does not understand the probationer's expression, it would be appropriate to stop and acknowledge and discuss the lack of understanding. At this time, similarities and differences in language style might also be discussed. It should be noted that such a situation offers a possibility of role reversal, for at this point in time, the probationer is the teacher and the officer is the learner. However, such a temporary shift in roles could well be repaid by a subsequently strengthened relationship. Using the probationer's "input" as a base, the officer would be well advised to do some informal research to reduce the gaps in verbal production and comprehension between him and the probationer. Needless to say, this is a non-verbal way of saying, "I care" and "I want to help." The time and the temporary sacrifice of role would be well spent, because it would result in the two communicants being able to "understand" one another and thus to arrive at the necessary congruence of goals for any rehabilitative effort to commence.

No dicussion of rehabilitative work with alienated and rebellious youth would be complete without some reference to the use of a group approach with these youngsters. Bearing in mind the high priority which adolescents give to peer associations and peer values, the probation officer could harness some of their natural, informal groupings to the goal of rehabilitation. Some youngsters who live in the same neighborhood, or who share the same interests, or who have similar problems could be seen together. Here, in a formal structure, the same kind of discussions that they have in their unstructured street corner gatherings could be utilized to constructive purpose. There is growing evidence that there is considerable "peer-therapy" in such groupings, and that, while an adolescent may be unable to work out his own problem, he is quite capable of helping another talk his through, gaining some self help in the process.[18] In addition, if the probation officer is able to gain the acceptance of such a group, his stature with the individuals in the group is enhanced and the rehabilitative work with each of them is furthered.

Summary

Alienated and rebellious youth constitute one of the central social problems of our time. Many of them become by definition delinquents. This paper has taken the position that the youngsters so labelled are essentially lower class youth who come from a "culture of delinquency" analagous to the "culture of poverty." Handicapped by family instability, poor housing, and generally low socio-economic status, these youngsters are alienated because they are unable to make timely adaptations to the change characteristics of a highly complex society. Unable to achieve in socially acceptable ways, they seek the standard ends of success by deviant means. They feel that no one really cares, so they adopt a facade of uncaring, hostility, and aggression.

In terms of rehabilitation, it has been suggested that the alienated must be convinced that it is worthwhile to care. This is the probation task, which the probation officer can achieve by increasing the probationer's self evaluation. It has been suggested that this can be achieved by restructuring the environment, where possible; and, in the supervisory relationship through (1) questioning as opposed to telling, (2) empathic response, (3) "cutting through" the facade to the probationer's basic feelings, and (4) by reaching out to the language system to facilitate open and candid communication. Finally, in recognition of adolescent behavior patterns, the group approach to rehabilitation has been suggested as worthy of serious consideration.

Notes

1. Hemmendinger, Miriam, "Sonnets From the Probation Department." *Crime and Delinquency*, Vol. 7, No. 4, October, 1961.

2. Brown, William Neal, "Alienated Youth." *Mental Hygiene*, Vol. 52, No. 3, July 1968.

3. Josslyn, Irene M., M.D., *Psychosocial Development of Children*. New York, FSAA, 1948.

   __________, *The Adolescent and His World*. FSAA, 1959.

4. Witmer, Helen L. and Ruth Kotinsky, New Perspectives for Research on Juvenile Delinquency. Washington, D.C. Children's Bureau, 1955.

5. Lewis, Oscar, Five Families. New York, Basic Books, Inc., 1959.

__________, Children of Sanchez. New York, Random House, 1951.

6. The Challenge of Crime in a Free Society, A Report by the President's Commission on Law Enforcement and Administration of Justice, p. 55-87.

7. Ibid.

8. Harrington, Michael, The Other America. Baltimore, Penguin Books, 1963, p. 173.

9. Hunter, David, The Slums--Challenge and Response. Glencoe, Ill., Free Press, 1964, p. 21-22.

10. Cohen, Nathan (ed.), Social Work and Social Problems. New York, NASW, 1964, p. 6.

11. Schorr, Alvin, Slums and Social Insecurity. U. S. Depart. of Health, Education and Welfare, 1963, p. 11-31.

12. Hollingshead, A., "Class Differences and Family Stability," in Stein and Cloward, Social Perspectives on Behavior. Glencoe, Ill., Free Press, 1958, p. 45.

13. Sexton, Patricia, Education and Income: Inequalities of Opportunity in Our Public Schools. New York, Viking Press, 1961.

14. Herriott, Robert E. and Nancy Hoyt St. John, Social Class and the Urban School. New York, Wiley, 1968.

15. Hunter, David, The Slums, p. 64. (see above).

16. The Challenge of Crime in a Free Society. p. 63 (see above).

17. Brown, William Neal, "These People . . . Who Are They?" Washington, D.C., Brookings Institution, 1962.

18. The New Jersey experiences at High Fields and Essex Fields are excellent examples of this approach.

Part V

Practical Applications

23. What is Homesickness?

by Herbert Strean

From Camping Magazine, April 1959, published by Galloway Corporation, North Plainfield, N.J. Reprinted by permission.

A camp season seldom terminates without a director or a member of his staff being faced with a youngster who is homesick. Since the term "homesickness" is now part of camp nomenclature, it may be fruitful to define the illness, ascertain its causes, and refine our procedures in handling the problem.

We, at Camp Ramapo-Anchorage, a camp serving emotionally disturbed youngsters, found ourselves using the term so loosely for so many children who presented difficulties in their camp adjustment, that we decided to take a closer look at the concept.

As we subjected the question to serious examination and carefully reviewed our cases of so called "homesickness," we found that no two situations were identical and each had to be handled differently according to its own characteristics. When Johnny cried hysterically, "I miss my mother and I want to go home," he was reacting to a different set of stimuli than Jean who kept her thumb in her mouth, sat by a tree and spoke in monosyllables, saying, "The food is no good. I'm going to vomit if I don't go back home."

Though we at Ramapo were dealing with emotionally disturbed children, we suspected our findings would be applicable to other settings. Perhaps less dramatically in other camps, homesickness always shows itself somewhere in the camp cluster and must be dealt with quickly. After completing our study, we found that the cure for homesickness is not to send the child home, but to help the child adjust to camp.

Though each child presented a unique set of circumstances, we found that most of these homesick children could fall under one of three categories.

1. Mama's Little Boy. Nine year old Frank presented a real problem. When his bunk mates wanted to play ball or go swimming he sat on his bed and exclaimed, "I'm not going. I hate it here!" Regardless of the activity, Frank refused to participate. Added to this, he was extremely uncooperative in all camp routines. He refused to make his bed, take his showers, or use respectable table manners. It seemed quite clear Frank was not going to be a group member, no matter what happened.

As staff members discussed Frank, it was evident he was a boy who had everything done for him at home by his parents. He wanted to recapture the same situation at camp and was extremely frustrated when he found certain things were required of him. His response was to balk.

Children with this type of background greet camp staffs every year. Indulged at home, they have no reason to take any initiative, because everything is done for them. They virtually say, "Do it for me. I'm only interested in myself. I don't care about anybody. If you don't treat me like my mommy does, I won't stay at your place."

Our first response to Frank is often an angry one. We say to ourselves, "Who does he think he is? The other campers are not like this. They enjoy themselves!" It is indeed helpful for us to realize our annoyed reaction, for this is just the response a Frank is trying to induce. He plans "if they really get to hate me, they'll send me home."

One of the most expedient methods we found to help a Frank is to meet him half way. To ignore him would only cause him to withdraw more. To argue with him would make him balk or out-wit us. To treat him as mother did at home would turn camp into a nursery school.

As we discussed the Franks that we had dealt with over the years, a plan evolved which when practiced proved extremely helpful. If the adult gives Frank just a little mothering, he'll respond. If we make a deal with him that we'll tie one shoe lace if he ties the other, we half appear like the mother to whom he is accustomed. He likes the adult for sensing how he feels. He will push hard on the saw in arts and crafts a day or two after we have worked diligently on his lanyard. A Frank will soon reward the understanding adult with more independent behavior. As our Frank said, "I'm the kind of horse that, if you bring me to water and stay with me, I'll really drink."

In short, for this very overprotected child, we do protect him for a period, and he thanks us by protecting himself.

2. Sick of Home. Into this category fall many children. Often, they are ones who are dumped at camp because they would interfere with family vacation plans. Sensing that they were sent away from home so camp will serve as an official baby-sitter, they have to retaliate. What better means for retaliation than to disrupt the family vacation plans and insist that Mother and Father come up to camp immediately and take them home?

These children are often considered outsiders in their own homes. They know no other position and become outsiders in camp. Frequently they feel that their siblings at home are getting some type of indulgence, while they, the mistreated, suffer at camp.

This child, who is so unsure of his status in his household, cannot relax away from it. He is always preoccupied with thoughts of "What's going on at home?" As Martin, a boy quite sick of his home said, "They're plotting against me while I'm gone. They like my sister better than me and they're being extra nice to her. I won't let this go on!"

Helping this child is not an easy task. He has to be encouraged to verbalize his angry feelings to an adult who will listen. Sometimes, this may be too difficult for him and we have to tell him how angry he is. In either case, he has to be provided with an arena to discharge his righteous indignation. When this occurs, half the battle is won. What better outlet is there for somebody who feels he does not count than to have an adult insist that what he has to say is very important? When Martin was offered this opportunity he remarked,

"You really care how I feel. Nobody else ever did."

Another method of helping a child who is "sick of home" is to give him a place in the camp family. Joe, a child who could not accept the fact that his brother was having a wonderful time in the Canadian woods with his parents, was made chairman of the committee to discuss an overnight trip at camp. He was chief of a crew of boys doing the same thing that his family was doing in Canada and worked alongside his counselor, joyfully exclaiming, "My brother is missing something!"

The child who is sick of home must be helped to get rid of his fever by discharging his anger. He should also be given a ranking position in the camp family.

3. "There Are Tigers Here!" Jane, an eight year old girl, wanted to go home the first minute she arrived at camp. She was terrified of everything from water front to nature area. "Please, please let me go home. That's all I want!" Jane pleaded.

Why such a frightened exclamation from a little girl? The reason--Jane had been told some tall stories about camp and was certain that she was in for a torturous experience. Her brother had told her that if she did not pass her deep water test she would be spanked, and that if she went on a hike in the woods tigers would eat her up. She had no way of knowing what would happen to her at camp. Her fantasies were not dispelled until the head counselor, together with a camper who "had been through the jungle," joined her on an exploratory hike and oriented her to every area of camp. Jane saw with her own eyes just what camp was like and what she could anticipate.

From Jane we can learn that many children who have never before attended a camp arrive with their luggage and false illusions. Both must be unpacked immediately.

We, at Ramapo-Anchorage, are mindful of the fact that other dynamic formulations may exist regarding the homesick child. Furthermore, there are helpful procedures for them too. Nonetheless, handling each homesick child one by one, and being aware of the causes behind the trouble, we have found it necessary to send a homesick child back to his home in the last several years.

24. The Age Game

by Mildred R. Newman and E. Mark Stern

From The Psychoanalytic Review, vol. 51, no. 2, Summer 1964. Reprinted by permission.

This article considers a new therapeutic approach to children's conflicts. It is based on the concept that regression is helpful in the treatment of the emotionally disturbed child. The technique itself, which is called "The Age Game," was conceived spontaneously by one of the authors in response to her own children's complaints about being ages four and five, respectively. She was fascinated by their verbalized wish to be babies.

> "Okay," she said, "let's play a game. You can be any age that pleases you, but you must be that age and if you want to be a baby, you must play like you are a baby. If you do anything which is not what a baby does, you are out."
>
> The older child said that she would very much indeed like to be an infant.
>
> "Okay," said mother, "come cuddle in my arms and we'll make believe that you are an infant."
>
> The child sat down on her mother's lap, cuddled up and said, "I am a baby only two weeks old."
>
> "Oh, what a darling baby! You are just lovely. How are you, baby?"
>
> "Fine," replied the five-year-old child, at which point, of course, it was explained that two-week-old babies cannot talk. They probably could coo and they might smile, but they just couldn't talk.

The game was used for a number of years as a diversion when moods seemed to need a little cheering. After a time the children realized how good it was to be their own true age.

This suggested a therapy of re-enactment of early wishes in children, where there is a need to get at an "itchy" area of trouble so that there may be growth instead of stagnation. It also seemed possible that it might be of some use in selective moments in the psychoanalysis of adults.

The significance of regression in child therapy has been widely recognized. Melanie Klein[6] reasons that normal and pathological regression causes "the re-emergence of early infantile sexuality." She attributes Oedipal fantasies to the very earliest stages of life, and uses these regressive traces in her treatment of children, directly interpreting the Oedipal situation in them. Paula Heimann,[5] in espousing the work done by Kleinian child analysts, makes the following observation: " . . . the analysis of children and adults (has) shown us that the most crucial contents of the Oedipus complex, and the most severe conflicts and anxieties, relate to the primitive impulses and fantasies which form the early states of the Oedipus complex."

Anna Freud[1] infers that the "child's neurotic reactions (remain) grouped around the parents who are the original objects of the pathogenic past." However, Sara Kut[7] describes the phenomenon of "regressed conflicts" which she feels are "repeated in the analysis with the therapist as the actual object, and only resolved and finally given up when these (are) interpreted."

It is our feeling that regression centers not so much about primary outside objects, but is basically an expression of the child's desire for mastery and a conflict-free existence. It is doubtful, in our minds, that children are as concerned with early fears as they are with ideal moments of peace experienced earlier. Even looking back at a difficult infancy, a child might recognize it as an age lived through. The most anxious part of being one's own age is the unpredictability of the future. To look back at a closed book is to know that it began and ended, which makes for the attractiveness of regressive fantasies. Allowing for the fact that the earlier years may be filled with pain, they still, nevertheless, have been dealt with and are past.

Regression to earlier ages is both a fact and a useful tool in psychotherapy. The analytic situation itself creates a climate for behavior characteristic of the most dependent stages in a person's life. The transference experience opens up vistas for the acting-out of early infantile experiences. The couch is not unlike the crib, where the baby is unable to see his mother on demand. It is often reported by patients that the very helplessness and dependency make for a total change in their view of their age positions. In fact, total reliance of the patient on the analyst is the core of the transference neurosis, recommended by Freud as a step toward rehabilitation. To recoup one's self from the transference neurosis is to regain one's age.

Considerable work employing regression has been done by workers in the field of psychotherapy with adult schizophrenics. Sechahaye[12] states that a thorough exploration "into the regressed effective stage is extremely important in the application of symbolic realization, for only in proceeding from the actual level of regression can real contact with the patient be established."

Searles[10] emphasizes that:

> to join the (schizophrenic) patient more and more often in mutually enjoyable plays on words, contributions of chaotically nonsensical verbalization and uninhibited flights of fancy (has helped restore) what was best and healthiest in the patient's very early relationship with the mother, and it is upon this kind of playful and unfettered interaction, historically traceable to the beginnings of verbal relatedness in the young child's life that the patient's gradual development of firm ego boundaries, and use of more logically organized, adult forms of thought and communications can be founded. The therapist learns, to his surprise, that there is a kind of chaos and confusion which is not anxiety provoking and destructive, but thoroughly pleasurable--the playful chaos which a mother and a little child can share, or which two little children can share, where mutual trust prevails to such a degree that there is no need for self-defensive organization. (p. 43)

Hypnosis also involves chronological retrogression. The subject becomes fixated to a helpless circumstance in which only the hypnotist has any real authority. His sense of adulthood becomes diminished in the hypnotic condition. Age regression techniques are used in order to arrive at information about early functioning which may be diagnostically or therapeutically helpful. However, in hypnotherapy, as in other techniques, regression is used as an aid to growth. To make the patient potent is to make the present possible.

Regression in psychotherapy, like the transference and the resistance, seeks to acquaint both analyst and patient with areas of expression not always accessible in other relationships. Jules Masserman[5] discusses channels of communication as a road to the understanding of various developmental clusters. For example, in the very young, the most prominent needs are for security and care. Most motives at these early ages are built upon such needs. After adolescence, however, there are fairly strong aggressive drives. Prestige and sexual gratification take on greater importance.

Masserman considers the different age levels as pathways to articulation. He alludes to the various forms of communication which may call up various age levels. The appeal to the "inspirational" and "patriotic" tends to waken a schoolage child. However, the fact that all ages respond to early childhood sentiments shows that no part of our developmental life ever gets completely lost.

Any therapy technique rests on making an individual aware of the rewards of being his own age. Regression, therefore, must always surface those drives within the individual which push forward. To be a child for some patients is inviting, because only during childhood was there any reward, no matter how meager. A brief case in point will help clarify the meaning of this concept:

Jane, now a mother of two young children, was invited to spend the weekend with her parents. Living at her parents' home are two brothers, both of whom are severely disturbed, and suffer from severe helplessness. Jane came back to the city after this weekend enormously despondent. She felt quite unable to cope with her own children and the demands for being a responsible mother. It became clear during the interview that Jane was acting out her own infantile aspirations. Her mother said, during the weekend, that she was too strong, and this created a barrier between them. Jane realized that there was no way of getting close to her mother except by being helpless and emotionally ill. Jane displayed characteristics befitting a youngster who had at least a possibility of deriving some affection from her mother.

Both of Jane's parents were apparently very indulgent to the weak members of the family. Only by weakness could they see themselves as strong. Jane's strength made it impossible for any chance of closeness. Therefore, Jane acted as if she were once again a little child. However, this didn't work out very well for her and she had to sullenly face the prospect of being an adult. The only help the therapist could provide, in addition to pointing up to her the acting out and what it meant, was to reassure Jane about the bittersweet components of being part of one's age group. It might actually mean that she would not have all of the affection she desired from her mother. However, it would insure that she would be a more capable mother and mate. It would mean that she would have to face the pains and pangs of responsibility, but it would insure her a sense of dignity and freedom.

This case illustrates the theme attempted in the age game. The yearning to return to the years of helplessness is probably indicative of the desire for some gratification which was then possible. Now it seems that there is a sense of aloneness and pain in facing one's existential plight. Being alone is the unfortunate consequence of being older. One becomes more aware of aloneness as the years go by and the necessity of separation from the all-caring mother is recognized. Troubling as this may seem, it is, by necessity, a step in self-realization and fulfillment. Ideally, to recognize one's aloneness involves new possibility and choices. The older child is no longer protected by mother, is in fact no longer one with the breast. If he is to have chums, he must do this by choice and effort. How comforting it would be to go back, but one soon learns that there is a price involved. The price is the sacrifice of one's intrinsic desire for freedom and autonomy. No regression can ever be so comforting as to be a final goal. Sternbach[14] hinted at some factors which contribute to the therapy of arrested ego development in children. The need for the therapist to wean and guide, a task which he states is essentially "one of upbringing, of training, of encouragement, education and socialization," is obviously based on the assumption that much of the disturbed child's inner core has never been given a chance to develop.

Remembering that the age game was an outgrowth of an informal play technique used by one of the authors with her children, we can now introduce it into the therapeutic arena. Two cases will be presented, treated separately by each of the authors. The illustrations are not so much to focus attention on a specific therapeutic tool as to suggest variations based on the same principles that may be useful to the child analyst.

Case One

Doris, a ten year old girl, suffered from a severe school phobia brought on after a weekend trip alone with her father. The terrors surrounding school attendance were based on a strong suspicion on Doris' part that if she attended school through the day, she would return to find her mother dead. Diagnostically, it was understood through traditional play techniques that Doris' fear was based on an unconscious hostility to her mother. Her anxiety reached a climax when she was alone with her father on a weekend vacation. If her "good" wishes to be with her father could come true her "bad" wishes to kill her mother could also come true.

Most of the "bad" feelings were on an unconscious level. The child was certainly not aware of her fears as such. Her relationship to her father was an extremely close one, in part because of his seductive mode of relating to his daughter. This created guilts in Doris which she was unable to allow herself to deal with. Not only her being a child, but her being frightened of her own sexual attractiveness to her father, destroyed any real impetus for growing. Growing, in a sense, would involve more danger.

No amount of cajoling or bribery could get Doris to return to class. It seemed out of the question to Doris to leave her mother. The therapist was concerned with the possibility that a breakdown might result if any pressures were brought to bear on the child to return to school. One day the therapist mentioned the age game, described it and invited Doris to join her in playing. Doris had a brother who was four years old, and the analyst was aware of Doris' wish to be as young as Tony. This, the therapist felt, would mean both that Doris could be more like her father, and also lose her terror-ridden feelings for her parents.

Doris initially seemed disinterested, but then asked if she might play the game after all, and expressed the feeling that it would be nice to be her four year old brother. The therapist discussed the rules with her. She told Doris that she could choose any age she liked, but that if she acted a different age, she would have to be excluded. The challenge to remain in the game became a motivating factor, making it possible for the child to put a great deal of feeling into her newly adopted role.

Doris decided that her first undertaking would be age four. She could now act like Tony. She wanted to play a card game and told the therapist that she was going to cheat, because it was perfectly permissible to cheat at age four. She drew pictures in a haphazard fashion typical of a child four years of age. She was obviously being gratified at this age level. First, she could feel identified with her father, and secondly, she felt freed from her conflict. She was excused from attending school as long as she decided to be age four, giving her a sense of rightness about her behavior.

After some sessions, she decided to be age six. It was apparent that she was learning to trust the analyst, whom she regarded as most helpful in providing the scenery and advantages of a four-year-old and six-year-old, respectively. She was also impressed by the fact that the analyst was consistent in the enforcement of the rules. Doris could, at both ages four and six, learn to face her fears about leaving her parents for any length of time. Six years old created slightly more anxiety than four, but still it was not ten, which was the most troublesome age of all. The six-year-old level seemed best suited to her future plans.

At the next session, she made no mention of the game. Instead she drew a picture of being on a desert island with her father. She was able, at this time, to talk more freely about her desire to be with her father. Both therapist and child were in a better position to discuss the realities of her non-attendance at school and other related problems. Soon school created no problems. She was able to leave her mother for long periods of time during the day. The direction of therapy became more verbal. The girl is now sixteen years old and has returned to the analyst on rare occasions to report.

Case Two

A seven-year-old boy was seen in therapy because of general behavior problems in school, which threatened to drop him from the rolls. At home he was rebellious, refused to go to bed at night, and when he finally did, invariably wet the sheets. Psychological evaluation pointed to retardation. This evaluation caused the school to discharge him on the basis of inability to learn.

Timmy approached therapy with an avid interest in the toys around the room. He was fascinated by a water fountain and loved to spend hours mixing paints and diluting them as he went along with more and more water. Interpretive material was introduced in relation to water and paint, and his joy in elimination. His mother was so heartbroken about Timmy's asocial behavior that she tended to discourage all play activity at home for fear that it was inappropriate to this age. The therapist made it quite clear that he could play with "messy" paint and water if he chose and that, in fact, he might like to pretend he was a little boy, a very little boy, who had the opportunity to wet his bed without being censured. The therapist enlisted the mother's cooperation. She was asked to extend the rules of the game to the home. This meant that if Timmy chose to be a certain age, she would be informed of this and Timmy would be expected to carry through at this age at home, with all the advantages and disadvantages his choice involved.

Timmy chose to be a little baby, who was permitted to speak only to tell the therapist his wishes. The therapist and Timmy spent some time going over the rules and deciding what a little baby could and could not do. For example, a little baby could go to the park, but he could not walk in the park--he would have to be carried. This brought many smiles to Timmy's face who looked forward to the prospect of being carried across the room to an area the therapist had designated as the park. Once he arrived at the park, he was not permitted to romp around and play, because he could not yet have learned how to walk. To this he agreed, not thinking at the time of the limitations but about the advantages of being carried as a baby is carried.

As we expected, Timmy was titillated with being pampered. He was even informed that if he wanted to urinate and defecate, he would do so in his trousers, since a change of trousers and underwear was available at the clinic. Timmy never took advantage of this permission, but insisted on being carried to the "park" and the "playground." However, he balked at the idea that he could not play when he arrived in the symbolic playground, but had to remain in one place. The therapist explained to him that he could not talk to him very much while at the playground, since the therapist could not expect a little baby to understand more than baby talk. After three sessions of playing at being a baby, and being denied related privileges at home Timmy decided that he would begin to break some of the rules. He was then informed that he could no longer be a baby but would have to choose another age.

He next decided to become an adult, like the therapist. At the same time he chose to be his mother's husband. His mother was separated from Timmy's father and Timmy was enthusiastic about filling his father's place. He began to try to talk like an adult. When riding the subway with his mother, after leaving the clinic, he would take her arm, look for a seat which she could occupy and be, all in all, very attentive. He was, of course, not permitted to play as a baby. If he did, the advantages of adulthood could be taken away, such as a bed hour as late as he chose, and as many portions of food as he wanted. He could no longer drink from a bottle, or be permitted to urinate in his pants. The therapist also told him that he would have to control wetting his bed, as this was typical for a younger child and not for an adult.

Timmy stopped wetting his bed at this point, a pattern which did not return as long as he was in treatment. His behavior at school began to improve. No appreciable change could be seen in his general intellectual development, and it remained doubtful whether he could actually succeed in a regular school. His mother was more inclined to value psychotherapy and more available for cooperative efforts. The therapist had to leave the country at this time and was forced to drop the case. There was no systematic follow-up, since the clinic felt Timmy was doing sufficiently well and he was not, therefore, assigned to another therapist. The therapist heard from Timmy's mother a few years later about resuming treatment, and a suitable referral was made.

Discussion

The age game is primarily acceptable to children precisely because it is both playful and serious. Participation in games is an underlying motivating factor in attracting the youngster to serious business about himself. Involvement in play makes it possible to reach back to feelings and actions of an earlier age. Verbalization itself frequently falls short of presenting a true picture of a child's desire because of the lack of safety words connote during childhood and early adolescence.

Both authors have employed the age game in some form with selected adult patients. Here it takes on the nature of role playing. The patient is encouraged to feel and act as he might have at an earlier stage of his life. He is encouraged to deal with the feelings and thoughts he had then. For example, a therapist might suggest that the patient spend a session or two talking and thinking as he might have on the day he first entered school. Sometimes the patient is asked to act out a condensed twenty-four hour period typical of the time he was a small child. Individuals are encouraged to keep with the age as best they can.

Others workers have used related techniques with adults. Ferenczi[3] expresses his gratitude to workers in child analysis for having inspired a "game" in his analysis of adults. He states:

> When you consider that, according to our experience hitherto, and to the premises with which we start, most pathogenic shocks take place in childhood you will not be surprised that the patient, in the attempt to uncover the origin of his illness, suddenly lapses into a childish or childlike attitude. [Ferenczi then asks:] Is there any advantage in letting the patient sink into the primitive state of the child? (p. 137) [He answers somewhat later in his paper:] The analyst's behavior is . . . like that of an affectionate mother, who will not go to bed at night until she has talked over with the child all his current troubles; large and small, fears, bad intentions, scruples of conscience, and has set them at rest. (p. 137)

Coleman and Nelson[2] in their "paradigmatic psychotherapy" in which "demonstration" rather than interpretation "often proved valuable in the conduct of the therapy of borderlines" state: "The patient is placed in the position of a growing child who is subject to the impact of many personalitites with their disparate temperaments and viewpoints." In acting out many contrasting roles for the patient, the therapist becomes a "paradigm of the world in which the patient must learn to move."

Sechahaye[12] and Searles,[10] mentioned above, are involved in prolonged games with their patients. Sechahaye in one case felt that she became "mama-therapist" to a "schizophrenic child." The careful interpretation of symbolic foods for mother's breasts became a restorative tool in the famous case of René.

Moreno[9] in the psychodrama of the patient's conflict helps recreate old situations with new methods of resolution.

A return to the past or past event is lived through again, but as in a sometimes optimistic dream, with more power and a more comfortable ending. In still another form Moreno had attempted to eliminate the "interpersonal resistance" in a case of a child who expressed nothing but extreme hostility and disdain for his mother. He had actresses play through experiences in his life, but the significant woman, rather than being a mother was a princess, then a queen--on to a college professor, a mayor's wife, a nurse and finally his own mother. The mother herself did not appear, however, until the therapy helped to "interpolate resistances." The actress who played the queen was asked by the therapist to become more aggressive or more like the child's mother.

In another context one of the authors[13] helped a patient reveal the lost child in herself and thus assisted in the recovery of a classical case of disassociation or "split personality."

In this context we have attempted to point up the value of a patient acting contrary to his age within the therapeutic experience. One is reminded of Whiting's[15] statement that "If a child were permitted by the rules of his culture to perform the roles of any status he wished (i.e., any envied status), the process of socialization might be quite different from what it is." (p. 121) Why the older child is denied the right to be what he wants, or the right to act like a baby when it would be most helpful to him goes beyond the scope of this paper. We have found that the age game helps restore some of these privileges.

The concept of game makes it clear that much of what is denied in ordinary social process is permitted in the game. Children denied the use of large quantities of money are allowed to speculate on huge real estate ventures in the game, "Monopoly." Adults who dress according to the custom of the community may enter a masquerade contest. But always rules govern these games. Bateson[1] comments that in play and fantasy the player must agree upon rules. Thus for a schizophrenic to talk in a "word salad" within the psychological frame of therapy, is, in a sense, not pathological. After they have ceased to play they are free to discuss the rules and modify them. Thus it is in the age game. The child (or adult) plays his adopted role as does the therapist. If the rules are broken, then they are discussed, and either agreed on for the next role or modified to a point where they become another form of therapy as in the case of Doris where talking and drawing a picture become the new game.

The age game becomes of value as the participants, i.e., patient and therapist, learn the many faceted value of emotional growth from it. Stern[13] found in his work with an older adolescent that growth did not mean extinguishing the child part of a borderline schizophrenic adolescent girl. Instead, he found that helping the personality appreciate the introjected child and using it when needed will allow for more effective growth than the rigid controls we are too well aware of in our culture. Bateson states that the patient "must learn that fantasy contains truth." (p. 50) Those who help their patients play the age game will learn that the baby in their individual psychodynamic structures has something important to say to the more grow-up portion of the personality.* If it is not permitted to have its say then a rage may flare within. The age game is no more than a recognition of the importance of areas of personal expression ordinarily discouraged by social norms. Or to use Whiting's[15] words, " . . . the adult role is to some degree a carry over of part of the child's role." (p. 124) Whether used in child analysis or adult therapy, the age game can be an aid to the growth and development of an enriched personality.

* Searles[11] highlights this point: "As the patient makes emotional contact with the various previously repressed areas of his past experience, bit by bit, he eventually reaches the realization that, despite all the years of illness, as one patient expressed it with great relief, 'I'm still myself.'" (p. 188).

References

1. Bateson, G. A Theory of Play and Fantasy. _Psychiatric Research Reports,_ Vol. 2, 1955, p. 39-51.

2. Coleman, M. L. and B. Nelson. Paradigmatic Psychotherapy in Borderline Treatment, _Psychoanalysis,_ Vol. 10, 1957, p. 28-41.

3. Ferenczi, S. Child Analysis in the Analysis of Adults. M. Balint, ed. Final Contributions and Methods of Psychoanalysis. New York: Basic Books, 1955, p. 126-142.

4. Freud, A. Indications for Child Analysis. The Psychoanalytic Study of the Child, Vol. 1, 1945, p. 127-149.

5. Heimann, P. A Contribution to the Re-Evaluation of the Oedipus Complex--The Early Stages. M. Klein, P. Heimann and R. Money-Kyrle, eds. New Directions in Psychoanalysis. London: Tavistock Publications, 1955, p. 23-28.

6. Klein, M. The Psychoanalysis of Children. London: Hogarth Press, 1950.

7. Kut, S. The Changing Pattern of Transference in the Analysis of an Eleven Year Old Girl. The Psychoanalytic Study of the Child, Vol. 8, 1953. p. 355-378.

8. Masserman, J. Principles of Dynamic Psychiatry. Philadelphia: W. B. Saunders Co., 1946.

9. Moreno, J. L. Psychodrama (2nd Revised Ed.). New York: Beacon House, 1946.

10. Searles, H. F. Schizophrenic Communications. Psychoanalysis and the Psychoanalytic Review, Vol. 48, 1961, p. 3-50.

11. --------. Phases of Patient-Therapist Interaction. British Journal of Medical Psychology, Vol. 34, 1961, p. 169-193.

12. Sechehaye, M. A. A New Psychotherapy of Schizophrenia. Translated by G. Rubin-Robson. New York: Grune and Stratton, 1956.

13. Stern, E. M. Mirror-Dialogue Approach to the Treatment of a Borderline Psychosis. Journal of Existential Psychiatry, Vol. 4, 1964.

14. Sternbach, O. Arrested Ego Development and Its Treatment in Conduct Disorders and Neurosis of Childhood. The Nervous Child, Vol. 6, 1947, p. 306-317.

15. Whiting, J. W. M. Resource Mediation and Learning by Identification. I. Iscoe and H. W. Stevens, Eds. Personality Development in Children. Austin: University of Texas Press, 1960, p. 112-126.